Good Goodbyes

Good Goodbyes

Termination in Therapy from Beginning to Ending

Second Edition

Jack Novick

Kerry Kelly Novick

ROWMAN & LITTLEFIELD
Lanham • Boulder • New York • London

Rowman & Littlefield
Bloomsbury Publishing Inc, 1385 Broadway, New York, NY 10018, USA
Bloomsbury Publishing Plc, 50 Bedford Square, London, WC1B 3DP, UK
Bloomsbury Publishing Ireland, 29 Earlsfort Terrace, Dublin 2, D02 AY28, Ireland
www.rowman.com

British Library Cataloguing in Publication Information available

Library of Congress Cataloging-in-Publication Data

ISBN 9781538195765 (cloth)
ISBN 9781538195772 (paperback)
ISBN 9781538195789 (ebook)

For product safety related questions contact productsafety@bloomsbury.com.

♾ ™ The paper used in this publication meets the minimum requirements of American
National Standard for Information Sciences—Permanence of Paper for Printed Library Materials,
ANSI/NISO Z39.48-1992.

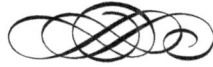

Contents

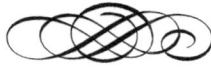

Acknowledgments

This is a book about endings, beginnings, and the work needed for a good goodbye. Part of this work is acknowledging the help received. We welcome this opportunity to do so.

Much of what we have learned has come from our patients, students, teachers, and colleagues. Traveling with them through the journeys of treatment, training, and mutual support has enriched our experience and our knowledge. We are grateful also for the many questions and ideas about ending treatment shared with us over the years.

Thinking deeply about what makes for a good clinical goodbye has helped us to recognize anew the developmental possibilities from treatment that can equip us all for the many partings and endings that life brings. As we approach the last period of our own lives, we think of our parents, Freda Novick and Harry Novick, Jeanne Kelly and Gene Kelly, Betsy Reisz and Karel Reisz, and our children and grandchildren, and rejoice in dedicating this book to them.

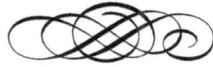

Preface

Since the publication of the first edition in 2006, there have been continuing fluctuations in professional attention to matters of termination of treatment in all modalities of clinical work. What has changed little, perhaps even worsened, are the rates of premature termination, failures of treatment, and avoidance of examination of causes. Herbert Schlesinger, a colleague who, like us, has maintained an interest in this topic, said in 2013 that ending seems to be the most difficult and the most important part of psychotherapy and noted that he had never known a conscientious psychotherapist who did not have trouble with endings.

Our experience with students over the years resonates with this, and the questions we addressed in the first edition are still relevant. In addition, many new factors seem to affect the fields of psychotherapy and psychoanalysis broadly and deeply, perhaps particularly and very visibly in the domain of satisfactory completion of therapeutic work. Social changes, the financial structure of health care, the continuing dominance of medication as an omnipotent cure-all, the possibility of online treatment, and many others raise new challenges and questions as we strive to offer effective treatment to alleviate human suffering and promote healthy development.

Students continue to grapple with termination, even as training programs offer little or no instruction or experience in thinking about it or in managing this critical passage. It is noteworthy that most psychoanalytic training programs no longer require a terminated case for graduation, while most psychiatric and psychology trainings allow annual turnover of patients or offer only short-term treatment modalities, thus giving students no experience of organic terminations. Their continuing questions have led us to generate this second edition, addressing both perennial and new issues in an effort to convey the importance of keeping termination in mind throughout treatment.

A word about us—how our background and training as psychoanalysts figure in this book. We think psychoanalysis offers the most comprehensive description of both the healthy and pathological development of the human personality. We practice and teach both psychoanalysis and what is called psychotherapy. We have found that our psychoanalytic training and experience have profoundly affected our psychotherapy work. We don't use different theoretical ideas or have different goals for patients, whatever the frequency of their treatment. In our work, in published accounts, and in reports from colleagues and students, we have seen intensive long-term cases that made little progress and once-weekly treatments that produced profound changes. Neither furniture nor frequency guarantees the outcome.

Psychoanalysis as a treatment method is intensive and usually long-term. This allows both patient and psychoanalyst the opportunity for a detailed study of the inner world of the person and space to practice alternatives and changes in the safety of the therapeutic relationship and setting. Each step of the process of change can be seen, and difficulties and resistances analyzed.

We think that the best training for doing psychotherapy is psychoanalysis. It was the first psychotherapy and is not a mysterious, arcane technique available only to the select few, either as practitioners or patients. If a baseball player is in a hitting slump, an examination of a slow-motion film of his swing allows for pinpointing the problem and correcting it. Similarly, experience of analysis and training in or study of such an intensive treatment modality is like having the slow-motion camera built into our minds and prepares the practitioner to do all kinds of treatment better. Psychoanalysis—as a theory, a general developmental psychology, and a clinical treatment method, with both clinical theory and technical precepts to offer—is the slow-motion, freeze-frame examination needed to make the best sense of phenomena. In this book, we draw from our experience of doing and teaching psychoanalysis and psychotherapy to offer all mental health workers our ideas about termination. We know that these ideas can be applied in all intensities and modalities of treatment. Therefore we will use the terms "analyst," "therapist," and "clinician" interchangeably throughout.

We are also "life-cycle psychoanalysts," always working with and looking at people's functioning through a developmental lens. In this book, we bring clinical examples drawn from work with patients of all ages.[1] Our aim is to expand the clinical repertoire, and there is much we can learn about the themes and issues of termination if we include work with children, adolescents, emerging adults, and their parents. Child and adolescent treatment remains a rich but still relatively untapped source of insight into therapeutic process and technique. Discussion of termination issues with younger patients is of value to those who work with that age group and also extends the technical options of those who work only with adults. Work with parents includes consideration of the challenges and rewards of adult development beyond parenthood. A full "life-cycle" emphasis includes the later adult phases as described by Erikson and other analysts.[2]

We write this preface after we have completed the manuscript of this second edition of *Good Goodbyes*. We are almost twenty years older than we were when the first edition was published. The usefulness to others of our ideas around termination has been heartening, and the continuing interest in further exploration and understanding that generated this second edition gives us hope for the future of therapeutic work that strengthens patients and clinicians in meeting life's challenges.

We are now old, in the last phase of our life cycle, and the exercise of rethinking termination has brought to mind the many goodbyes one experiences in a lifetime, as well as the last goodbye that will end this phase of life for us. It has also reminded us of the wellspring of emotional muscle that comes with thinking, doing, and sharing ideas, and we are happy to hold that endeavor in common with our colleagues, students, friends, and families.

We hope the second edition proves useful to old and new readers and that the additional bibliographic resources and tables are helpful.

Notes

1 A word about clinical examples and confidentiality—description and discussion of clinical work is a major modality of teaching and learning in our field, and yet respecting the privacy and confidentiality of patients' material is deeply important

on multiple levels. We address this at each stage of interaction with patients. From the start we assure patients that we will respect their privacy and not share details of their personal stories with anyone else; this is particularly salient for children and adolescents, where we are also doing concurrent parent work. We also state the exception to this practice, when the safety of the patient or anyone else is threatened, since actions, unlike thoughts or feelings, are public. In the working arrangements we agree to with each patient, we include their permission for anonymized/disguised material to be used for teaching and research, thus allowing for discussion of this issue from the beginning. In joint publications, we add a further layer of confidentiality by not identifying which of us was the treating clinician. And, in editing two casebook collections of clinical work and commentary, authorship was further anonymized by listing contributors' names at the beginning, but not identifying particular cases with any specific author. For further discussion of these issues, see D. Barrett and J. Miller (2024).

2   Erikson (1950); Pearl King (1980); Colarusso and Nemiroff (1979); Colarusso (2024); Novick, J. and Novick, K.K. (2016).

1

Introduction and Overview

Why Is a Process of Ending/ Termination Important?

Life is filled with hellos and goodbyes. In this book, we will talk about how the ending of treatment can be an opportunity to address these life tasks in new ways that lead to growth and change. Learning how to say a good goodbye strengthens a person's lifelong capacity to engage with separation, loss, and transformation. A good goodbye encompasses the mixture of feelings that inevitably accompanies change.[1]

Termination themes are the thoughts, feelings, and dynamics in both therapist and patient that relate to change, transitions, and endings. When we keep termination themes in mind from the very first contact, we are able to track progress throughout treatment. Eventually, as we shall describe in this book, this effort contributes to setting treatment goals, revising and adding to them as treatment proceeds, keeps the therapy moving, and helps patients consolidate the insights gained, integrate new coping mechanisms and patterns of relating, and synthesize the changes they have experienced. Recognizing and practicing these positive changes is crucial for the client's long-term well-being and continued personal growth.

How Has Termination Been Understood in the Past?

For the first fifty years of the twentieth century, psychoanalysts had little to say on the topic and were rather cavalier in the way they dealt with termination. However, after a series of mid-century symposia by British, American, and French analysts, termination became a topic of interest and investigation, especially in the United States.[2] Articles, reports, and books on termination appeared with increasing frequency. Engagement with the topic seemed to reach a peak in the 1990s. At that point, there was general agreement that there is a distinct phase of treatment that can be designated the termination phase.

This was soon followed by an emerging tendency to downplay or deny the importance of termination. Analysts began to question the need to set a date, to ask whether too much emphasis was being put on the topic, and to suggest that a distinct termination phase need not be differentiated.

A significant dimension of the confusion around termination in the field derives from the fact that therapy students do not go through the same experience of termination that their patients do. Psychodynamic clinical training usually requires students to enter treatment. A "training analysis" bears little relation to ordinary psychotherapy or psychoanalysis, because the motivation for treatment is different, the conditions of confidentiality are potentially compromised, and especially because neither party is likely to have to say goodbye at the end, since their relationship will be changed into one of collegiality. Despite attention to this problem from the 1930s on, many psychoanalysts continue to deny this glaring difference, perhaps contributing to the neglect of attention to termination.[3] We will consider more about the impact of this difference in the chapter on termination.

What New Model of Termination Are You Proposing?

In his classic book on technique, Edward Glover emphasized that the only rule is that there are no rules.[4] We all accept that each treatment is a unique relationship between two individuals, which takes place at a particular cultural, social, and historical time. Much of what transpires between the two may be paraverbal and therefore unknown or even unknowable. A particular therapy cannot be replicated, and this may make it more of an art than a science, challenging our capacity to make general observations and devise comprehensive technical approaches.

But we can look for observable commonalities in how treatments unfold, as well as in how they go awry or end badly. "Termination" has usually referred only to the final phase of therapy, when the active part of the therapeutic relationship comes to an end. For purposes of learning, teaching, and the conduct of treatment, psychotherapy or psychoanalysis can be broken down into evaluation, beginning, middle, pretermination, termination, and post-termination phases. In practice, there is not such a clear demarcation between phases; they are not like stops along a railroad line. Common themes, issues, conflicts, and affects thread throughout each treatment. However, particular themes and tasks are highlighted at different times as treatment progresses, and they can be conceptually organized in terms of phases. This heuristic device allows us to sharpen our focus on termination phenomena as they appear.

Psychodynamic theory and understanding provide multiple vantage points—each of the metapsychological points of view, different levels of development, different technical dimensions, to name a few.[5] We can examine the whole process of treatment from the vantage points of transference, defense, therapeutic alliance, object relations, the tasks of each phase of treatment, and so forth, since it has been established that each of these aspects is part of therapy throughout and each can illuminate different aspects of the personality.

As we move into the technical chapters of this book, we will organize the material by phases, considering the therapeutic alliance tasks of each phase that challenge client and therapist to respond, and we will consider what elements of termination themes, both positive and risk factors, both open- and closed-system aspects, can be discerned and addressed.

Contrary to the opinion that termination is only relevant at the end, if at all, we will consider the whole treatment from the vantage point of termination phenomena in each phase from the very first contact. Looking through the lens of termination can particularly highlight past, present, and future issues around saying goodbye, separation, autonomy, loss, and attachment.

We will demonstrate in this book the positive utility of attention to termination throughout treatment, since experience demonstrates that a bad ending can ruin a good therapy or even lead to physical illness or death.[6] Lack of a thorough familiarity with the large array of themes, issues, obstacles, criteria, and phenomena of termination in psychoanalysis and psychotherapy may lead to the waste of a great amount of precious time, effort, and money, with little benefit to the patient, the therapist, or the field of mental health.[7] Martin Bergmann stated in 1996 that "no paradigm of termination has been made part of the professional equipment of the psychoanalytic practitioner."[8]

What Needs to Be Included When Thinking about Termination?

We think about overarching models of development and functioning that offer treatment goals that apply to all patients. We are particularly inspired by one of Freud's stated goals for analysis. In *The Ego and the Id*, Freud said, "Analysis does not set out to make pathological reactions impossible, but to give the patient's ego *freedom* to decide one way or the other."[9] Nearly fifty years later, Rangell reiterated that the goal of analysis is choice.[10] Neither author spelled out the alternative possibilities in detail, a choice between what and what?

In this book, we propose a new model for thinking about termination and working with termination themes throughout treatment. This new technical model rests on our evolving ideas about two systems of self-regulation.

What Are the Two Systems of Self-Regulation?

From earliest infancy, everybody needs to feel safe, that their world is predictable, that their experience is encompassable, and that obstacles can be overcome, problems can be solved, and conflicts resolved. If the method the growing child generates is based on competent, effective interactions with the important people in their world, in the context of mutually respectful, pleasurable, and loving relationships formed through realistic perceptions of the self and others, they will be able to remain open to inner and outer experiences and cope creatively with life's challenges.

If overwhelmed by repeated experiences of helplessness, pain, despair, abandonment, violence, or other terrible circumstances, people at any age may turn away from reality, feeling that safety resides in a magical world of omnipotent solutions, in which the individual has a conscious or unconscious belief in real power to control others, hurt them, force them to submit to one's desires. Such a learned response to painful or negative interactions with caregivers or other adverse experiences can come to feel like the most dependable safeguard and take on an addictive quality, restricting the person's attempts to try other solutions and pathways to problem-solving and conflict resolution.

Our clinical work with patients of all ages has led us to think that clinicians can benefit from a model of development that describes in more detail two distinct kinds of solutions to conflicts as the person faces the internal and external challenges of each phase in life. Our two-systems model of development describes two possible ways of responding to feelings of helplessness. One system of self-regulation is attuned to inner and outer reality, has access to the full range of feelings, and is characterized by competence, love, and creativity. We call this the "open system."

The other, which we call the "closed system," avoids reality and is characterized by power relations, omnipotence, and stasis.[11] This omnipotent, sadomasochistic system is closed, repetitive, and increasingly resistant to change. In a distorted personality development, it can become a structure regulating feelings of control, safety, excitement, enjoyment, power, and self-esteem.

Through the longitudinal development of open and closed systems, with potential choices available at each phase throughout life, we may see the open-system effort to transform the self, making use of inner and outer resources, in contrast to the closed-system aim to control, force, and change others. Elucidating the operation of these two systems in the treatment relationship offers patients a genuine choice about how to live their lives.[12] A summary table can be found at the end of this book.

At the outset of treatment, it is the therapist who can use the idea of two systems of self-regulation to carry the conviction of the eventual potential of choice. The knowledge of open-system possibilities, manifested in the tasks of the therapeutic alliance that the analyst initiates with the patient, is what lends the therapist courage and hope to venture into the patient's "borderland"[13] to guide both people to the possibility of choice. From the beginning of therapy, the analyst keeps in mind the treatment goal of the possibility of greater open-system functioning, and this is part of what moves the treatment along toward a good ending. We can assess interventions throughout treatment in terms of whether and how they give the patient expanded possibilities of choice and change.

Here are examples of how some patients talked about choice at the end of their treatment:

> Mr. M said, "It's my life. I have only one life, and I have to choose. It's hard to admit that I was wrong, hard to admit that my pain buys me nothing but aspirin. But then I never knew that I had a choice, that I could choose to live a real life with real pleasures and real love."
>
> Mr. Z said, "I'm struggling with my disappointment in you, in me, and in the analysis. You're not perfect, and the analysis didn't turn me into the perfect, all-powerful person I always expected to be. I can feel the pull, but if I go there, I'll have to destroy all the hard work, the good work we did to help me be more settled and happy in my skin, in my home, in my life. I now have a choice. For that, thanks."

The two-systems model has also been applied to political systems, biology, cognitive processing, and many other categories of belief and behavior.[14] We can now recast the overarching goal of treatment and what we assess for termination as the restoration of the capacity to choose freely between open and closed systems of functioning and self-regulation.

What Are the Types of Termination?

It is important to note first that the majority of terminations are premature, especially in child and adolescent work. We wonder if that fact contributes to a general reluctance to study the topic. Nevertheless, understanding the determinants and characteristics of each type of termination can equip us to address them appropriately.

Premature Terminations Initiated by One Party Alone

Forced

Here, the decision is prematurely arrived at and initiated by the analyst. This may be due to relocation, illness, pregnancy, or death. Or, as is often the case, a termination is forced by the therapist as the result of countertransferences and counter-reactions to the patient.

Unilateral, Premature End Initiated by the Patient

There is a range of factors at work here. There can be seemingly valid external reasons, such as geographic moves or physical illnesses. Often, however, there are intense resistances to change and growth. There may be avoidance of legitimate or transferential negative feelings about the analyst, or the acting out of an unanalyzed negative therapeutic motivation.[15]

The exponential impact of social media usage has given rise to both a term and a normalization of a particularly hostile form of unilateral rupture in interactions and relationships, that is, "ghosting." We will consider technical responses to this pattern in subsequent chapters.[16]

Unilateral, Premature End Precipitated by Parents or Significant Other

As we will describe in subsequent chapters, parents struggle with many different feelings about their child's treatment. Dynamic concurrent parent work can often address these and protect against unexpected or abrupt treatment terminations. Significant others in an adult patient's life can also interfere with or undermine a treatment and precipitate a premature ending.

Interminable

Patient's Contribution

Some treatments take a long time because the problems are complex, and the patient has organized his personality to maintain himself in the face of intense difficulties. This is different from an entrenched refusal to terminate, signs of which can be picked up from the very beginning if the therapist knows what to look for. A patient's difficulty or refusal to progress becomes evident as treatment proceeds, and the problem becomes acute with prolonged resistance to entering the pretermination phase of treatment. Fear of open-system functioning and enmeshment in closed-system sadomasochistic relationships, played out in the treatment, are critical factors in maintaining interminable therapies. Schlesinger discussed the importance of spotting a turning point in treatment when there is a shift in the needs being met; Salberg described many cases where those needs continued to be gratified instead of analyzed.[17]

Therapist's Contribution

We will spell this out in greater detail later, but an unduly prolonged treatment can hinge on the therapist being pulled into a relationship of enthrallment with the patient, a joint search for impossible perfection or union, part of a closed-system solution to conflicts and anxieties. Premature termination or prolonged therapy are dangers at each phase of treatment. We will describe and discuss how to recognize and prevent these at different phases.

Pause or Intermittent Treatment

Many child therapists have described situations in which it seems appropriate to stop a child's treatment for the time being, as there has been a developmental consolidation at a new phase. If the challenges of a subsequent phase or circumstances once again overwhelm the child's ego, treatment can be resumed and continued to a point of genuine termination. With adolescent patients in particular, the analyst can maintain a link with the patient by suggesting a pause, rather than accepting the patient's unilateral termination plan. We think that these lessons from child and adolescent analysis may be usefully applied in adult work.

Mutually Agreed on Termination (MAT)

Here, both patient and clinician come to the conclusion that the patient has changed significantly, and progressive movement is evident. A pretermination phase starts in order to strengthen forward movement, analyze resistances to ending, and determine what can be addressed in a termination phase. MAT is a goal for the setting of the termination date, but the pattern of mutuality, the construction of a partnership or alliance, is worked on from the first contact.

In order to avoid the issues surrounding a forced termination, many clinicians now use the phrase "mutually agreed termination" in case reports. However, calling an end mutual does not necessarily make it so. Mutuality is a therapeutic alliance goal from the very beginning and not something that can be tacked on to the end like a magical blessing or a surprise dessert. We have heard many cases where the decision was premature or decided unilaterally by one person or the other, then called a "mutually agreed" decision as a face-saving gesture.

How Does Attention to Termination Relate to Treatment Goals?

The overarching goal of treatment is restoration to the path of progressive development, with open-system choices available for problem-solving and conflict resolution. Each phase of treatment can elucidate and contribute a particular component to that goal.

From a termination perspective, the long-range goal of treatment is open-system post-termination living. Therapy is not an end in itself. The medium-range goal is to proceed through the phases of treatment and consolidate open-system ego achievements. The short-range goals of treatment refer to the specific tasks of each phase, the elucidation of pathological interferences to competent ego functioning, and the enhancement of ego functions, open-system self-regulation, and positive affective experiences, past and current.

How Do We Use Material from Child and Adolescent Treatment in Our Model of Termination?

In this book, we use clinical examples drawn from work with patients of all ages. Termination evokes deep and universal feelings for everyone, rooted in all stages of development. We can look back from adult experience to reconstruct earlier history (what psychoanalytic metapsychology characterizes as the genetic point of view), and we can look forward from infant, child, and adolescent experience to discover what remains important (the developmental point of view). A life-cycle approach also includes the challenges and rewards of all phases of adult development.

Notes

1 As Schlesinger noted in his volume on termination, "Loss is the single universal and essential human experience." He also said, "Without the ability to experience loss it is not possible to experience gain." 2013, pp. 391–392.

2 Symposium 1950.

3 A. Freud 1968 [1938]; Milner 1950; Greenacre 1971; J. Novick 1997; Craige 2002, 2009; Schlesinger 2005, 2013; J. Novick and K.K. Novick 2006; Kantrowitz 2015.

4 E. Glover 1955.

5 K.K. Novick and J. Novick 2002.

6 From Freud's Wolf Man on, the history of analysis is filled with cases of mishandled terminations (1918). This is what happened to a number of the analytic cases reported by Firestein (1978). A theory of catastrophe following mishandled terminations has been elucidated in the work of Kinston and Cohen (1988, 1990). In Heather Craige's groundbreaking survey and interview study of recent graduates of psychoanalytic institutes, 28 percent admitted to intense disappointment in their analysis (2002). In a later paper, Craige presents numerous moving accounts of how even a seemingly successful analysis can be ruined by a mishandled termination (2009). Kantrowitz found that 59 percent of the clinicians treated psychoanalytically in her sample ended with a premature termination, either forced by the analyst or unilaterally initiated by the patient (2015).

7   For a fuller discussion of the many historical resistances and obstacles to understanding and studying termination phenomena and techniques, see J. Novick 1997.

8   Quoted in J. Novick, 1997, p. 172. In the current climate of clinical training in various disciplines, most students graduate without experience of a terminated case. We and Schlesinger (2013) both emphasize that termination issues should be taught about from the inception of clinical work. Otherwise qualified clinicians are left without training or personal experience for the conduct of a planned termination when they begin practice.

9   Freud 1923, p. 50 note; our italics.

10   Rangell 1982.

11   J. Novick and K. K. Novick 1991, 1996a, b, 2002, 2016; K. K. Novick and J. Novick 1998.

12   Clinical work is the database for our two-systems model. There are recent descriptions of two-systems models of regulatory functioning at neurological, physiological, and cellular levels from research science in allied fields. For further discussion of the possible links between these convergent approaches to epigenetic development, see Singletary 2024, 2020.

13   Hughes 1884.

14   See, for instance, Fromm 1947; Mayr 1988; von Bertalanffy 1968; Rokeach 1960, 1951; Hoffer 1951; Adorno et al. 1950. It is noteworthy within the arena of psychodynamic theoretical models that the two-systems perspective is useful and relevant across different schools of thought and their technical implications (Donner 2019). It carries useful analogs also to the empirical work on categories or modes of attachment (A. Freud 1965; Bowlby 1969, 1980; Ainsworth 1985, 1991; Ainsworth et al. 1991; Sroufe 2020).

15   J. Novick and K.K. Novick 2007 [1980].

16   Norcross et al. 2017. This research on how people have ended therapies of all kinds described ghosting as "not the most productive way" (quoted in NY Times 10/27/23). Norcross noted that, when people leave abruptly or avoid the difficult work of saying goodbye, they may be repeating the avoidant, non-assertive behavior that brought them in.

17   Schlesinger 2005; Salberg 2010.

2

Evaluation/Exploration

What Can You See at Evaluation That Is Relevant to Termination?

At the evaluation phase, along with the many other aspects explored, it is important in relation to termination to discern issues that might lead the patient to end treatment unilaterally or prematurely or to push the therapist to reject the patient and force a termination. Equally, we listen for strengths that will support the patient through difficult times, including separations and the eventual ending of treatment.

How Can You Identify and Address Both Risk and Protective Factors for Termination During Evaluation?

Good Feelings/Feeling Good

Keeping in mind the overarching goal of movement from closed-system to open-system functioning, we are alert to and actively inquire about instances in the patient's life of joyful, creative functioning and loving, differentiated relationships. We continue the assessment until we can discern what Sroufe, on the basis of his attachment research, so eloquently called "islands of positive earlier experience."[1]

A pretty, bright young woman came to see me for a first appointment. Miss Q talked about friends who would "do absolutely anything" for her, yet she felt she couldn't really talk to them. She couldn't be more specific about her unhappiness, and she described a healthy, uneventful childhood and pleasant relationships with parents and siblings. I was disposed to like Miss Q on the basis of my first impression but felt stymied and baffled when she dumped her ill-defined problem in my lap. A potential dynamic was being set up: she would be the miserable one, and she would get me to be the one with the magical omniscience to fix it. My discomfort at our being cast in these roles spurred me to think about an alternative approach that would move us toward the possibility of a more open interaction. I asked her when in her life she had felt wonderful.

Miss Q looked puzzled, shrugged, and said, "With successes." When I asked for specific instances, she perked up and told me with a shining face about a serious athletic pursuit in her adolescence, when she had excelled and won many competitions. Her face fell, however, when she said, "But then there were the bad times when I didn't win, and they canceled out the good ones." I remarked on what an interesting paradigm she had just described, that it would be important for us to look at how it worked— that if the bad times canceled out the good ones, she was left with nothing. We talked more about her indeterminate feeling of unhappiness possibly relating to a difficulty in holding and accumulating good feelings inside. We had begun together to see the outlines of an internal conflict over pleasure, and understanding this could be defined as a goal of therapy.

The pain and distress that bring a person to a therapist are often what is first presented and, because therapists are skilled at listening, empathizing, and absorbing these feelings, we may focus only on those difficulties, missing an opportunity to demonstrate to the prospective client that we are interested in their whole selves. The belief that pain is the most reliable way to get attention, connection, and needs met is often an organizing aspect of closed-system functioning. When we keep in mind the idea that we want eventually to be able to move forward with the patient to broader-based relating, we are protecting against unduly prolonged treatments.

The therapist needs to find evidence during the evaluation of open-system capacities or possibilities in order to have conviction that the patient will eventually be able to access and develop these potentials of their personality.

> Mr. G's wife had threatened to leave him unless he sought treatment. He presented a list of abusive behaviors with bravado and a barely concealed challenge to me to reprimand him. Instead, I focused on the essential needs served by his behavior, adding that everyone has these same needs. Mr. G seemed a little flustered by my comment but then recovered by saying that he knows how to get what he needs without asking favors of anyone. I then asked Mr. G. to tell me about his wife. After some initial grumbling about her being unfair, oversensitive, and deserving of his abusive behavior, he began to talk about her in a softer tone with admiration for her achievements. I said to Mr. G that, despite the fact that he was so hard on his wife, he also seemed to value the relationship. Mr. G began to cry and said he felt she was an essential part of his life, that he needed treatment in order to keep her. With access to Mr. G's open-system love for his wife, there was potential for making a recommendation that Mr. G begin an analysis and articulating a shared goal in terms of internal change.

In relation to looking at open-system self-regulation in the patient at the time of evaluation, we have found that it is important to have a long enough period to discern areas of past and current functioning that point to achievements, talents, moments of joy and love, and possibly even genuine satisfaction in the process of work and creativity. General training practice is to assess prospective patients in only one or two sessions. We often spend much longer in the exploratory/evaluation phase and find that it increases the rate of acceptance of treatment recommendations. We seek to know where and when the patient experiences pleasure and whether it can be maintained. Often, pointing out to the prospective patient his or her difficulties in experiencing ordinary pleasure or satisfaction provides a crucial initial motivation and defines an important shared goal of treatment.

History of Separations, Losses, and Leave-Taking

We ask about separations throughout the person's life, as it is well-established that early separations, abandonments, and losses can have profound lifelong effects that will emerge in relation to small and large interruptions in treatment, including termination. We want to know how the person has left different situations and relationships in the past. This alerts us to patterns of ending that the patient might reproduce in treatment.

> Mr. H, a middle-aged man, sought treatment for depression. As he described his childhood, he mentioned how he had always been advanced in his studies, skipping grades and starting the next stage early. From this information, I pointed out that there was a pattern of never having to go through a leave-taking, never having time for a proper goodbye, and suggested that it might be important for us both to be alert for a repetition of this pattern in our work together and in other relationships.

How Did They Leave Home as an Adolescent?

Separations and losses are there from the very beginning of life, and modes of attachment begin to develop equally early. These affect all subsequent experiences of separation and changes throughout life, but become consolidated at adolescence. Unilateral terminations by adults often reflect their adolescent style of leaving home.[2]

> Thirty-five-year-old Mr. E entered treatment suffering from suicidal depression and a life-threatening disease. For some time, we struggled with both the reality and the fantasy of impending death; gradually he emerged from this psychically induced life-threatening situation. He shed excess weight, his hypertension improved, he was no longer depressed or suicidal, and he regained his capacity to work and to love. Increasingly, however, he became passionately involved in airplane flying. As he continued to improve, he informed me one day that he would have to stop treatment because he was using the money he had set aside for therapy to subsidize his flying lessons.

Only when I inquired whether his enthusiasm for flying was something new or the rekindling of an old passion did the patient say that he had become preoccupied with motorcycles as an adolescent. One day, he had precipitately taken all his college money out of the bank and left home, riding away on his motorcycle, never to return. He then laughingly remarked that the airplane was probably his motorcycle.

In this example, we can see the impact of omitting to find out in the evaluation what the adolescent pattern of leave-taking had been. It is important to bring this into the shared knowledge of patient and therapist as soon as possible. With this information known between them, the patient and therapist can set goals for treatment in relation to leaving.

Patients' Fantasies and Expectations about Treatment

We listen for the patient's fantasies about treatment or the therapist and the patient's ideas about how long treatment might last; these constitute the *patient's treatment plan*. The pioneer psychoanalysts Ferenczi and Rank emphasized the importance of analyzing the conditions and requirements that patients associate with the end of analysis.[3] If this is not attended to throughout, it can defeat the final result of the treatment, no matter how well it is carried out beforehand. Large-scale studies of psychotherapy find a significant correlation between the patient's expectation about the length of treatment before the start and the actual duration of treatment.[4] This effect is powerful enough to cut across class, sex, and age. Most patients enter treatment with their own conscious or unconscious unilateral treatment plan; unless we make this an explicit object of investigation, the patient's unilateral plan can become confused with a genuine termination and will even take precedence over a successful termination.

Everyone has experienced separation, abandonment, rejection, or loss at some point. People often start treatment anticipating further loss and may use a variety of means to defend themselves: at one extreme, they may imagine total dependency, where neither can leave; at the other, they aim for complete solipsistic self-sufficiency. This is a built-in fundamental ambivalence. From the very start of therapy, these forces may become manifest in the patient's treatment plan: a struggle between the wish to terminate prematurely or to turn treatment into an interminable situation.

Many patients who have a sophisticated intellectual understanding of the process of treatment start with the announcement that they are "not going to have transference feelings." Others may state or indicate that they will never leave, saying, "You're stuck with me," or, "If I just stay long enough, I can force you to be the mother I have always wanted."

One idea that is often quite conscious from the start is an idealized view of the therapist. A patient can come for evaluation citing many past failed treatments and expressing the expectation that this new therapist will be the one who can succeed where others have failed. Gratifying though this may be to the clinician, this is an invariable marker of a potential externalizing, controlling, and sadomasochistic relationship.[5] If we explore this idealized expectation, we can begin to differentiate a doomed, magical, omnipotent attribution from realistic and nurturing hope.

Why Is Sadomasochism Important in Relation to Termination?

Personalities organized around sadomasochistic fantasies, power relationships, and the omnipotent beliefs underlying them are highly resistant to change and movement forward. This closed-system pathology will, therefore, interfere with restoration to the path of progressive development and contribute to resistances that may be demonstrated by premature, unilateral termination, stalemate leading to the therapist actively forcing the end of treatment, or prolonged, interminable treatment. Closed-system organization of the personality has served important and legitimate needs for the patient, often for many years. Given the security, safety, and gratification that omnipotent beliefs provide to the individual, it is indeed questionable why anyone would give it up. What is the alternative? The patient fears that the only alternative is the experience of helplessness, rage, or traumatic guilt that originally gave rise to the defensive omnipotent delusion.

When Will Treatment End?

All patients have concerns about the length of treatment. In work with parents of child and adolescent patients, instead of automatically assuming that practical and logistical issues necessarily constitute resistances to treatment recommendations, we have found that it is important to acknowledge the realistic demands that therapy makes of families. With that respectful, shared open-system discussion, it then becomes possible to look further into parental fantasies about treatment and their fears that treatment will go on forever.

With this access, we begin to generate termination criteria. Rather than constricting the work by giving parents a specific time estimate, which may rapidly become their unilateral treatment plan, we describe restoration to progressive open-system development as the goal. This will be seen in the child's acceleration of forward development, in a renewed pleasure in their own functioning, and in the establishment of a positive, sturdy parent-child relationship. This is an accessible and logical development from earlier discussions of symptoms and anxieties as interferences to progressive development. With these termination criteria in mind, parents and therapist are set to work together to monitor areas where progress has resumed and those where there is still little movement.[6] We think this approach to evaluation is equally effective in working with adults. Here, too, we tend to extend the evaluation longer than is the usual practice, and, as with Mr. G above, we try to work until we have established the beginning of a shared understanding of conflict and the goal of making open-system functioning available.

What Is Gained from Talking about Termination at the Very Beginning?

Inclusion of these termination criteria from the very beginning is a further application of the model of two systems of self-regulation. Establishing the description of progressive development in terms of growth in open-system functioning allows us to note the contrast with parents of child patients when closed-system functioning persists or reappears. Continuation and maintenance of the treatment then make sense to parents. Equally, for patients of all ages, the movement from closed-system pain and stasis to open-system competence, pleasure, love, and creativity as a goal of treatment makes sense and takes away some of the mystery and fear of starting treatment.

Are There Other Reasons to Complete Evaluation before Beginning Therapy?

The recommendation, setting the frame, and discussing the working arrangements are part of the end of the evaluation phase. We have found that there is a series of issues that is often elided, dismissed as merely business-related, and not as important as the emotional and psychological issues that represent the content of the work.

What Impact Do Administrative Aspects of Therapy Have?

Our experience has been that relegating the business, or "nuts and bolts," to a lesser position generally serves defensive needs in either the therapist or the patient. Many therapists confuse being liked, or establishing rapport with prospective patients, with avoiding making any reality demands in the treatment relationship. This can hold true when arrangements are made with an adult patient or with a child or adolescent patient's parents. If we do not clearly define the working arrangements, it leaves open the potential for having a real-life negative impact on the therapist, rather than keeping the patient's or parents' anger and inevitable hostility in the safe arena of thoughts and wishes to be understood and addressed.

An example from supervision is the case of a sixteen-year-old whose father was highly competitive with everyone, including his daughter's male therapist. In meetings with the therapist, he had nothing but criticism and denigrating comments. It was difficult for the therapist to deal with his own counter-reactions in a constructive way. The therapist neglected to tell his supervisor what the billing arrangements were, beyond saying that he arranged payment in his usual way. He billed for the past month on the first of the next month and didn't specify a deadline for payment. This left a lot of room for confusion and invited acting out. The father took advantage of this vague arrangement and tended not to pay until the very end of the next month. Before the therapist realized what was happening, the father was behind many months, and soon the bill mounted to thousands of dollars. The therapist found it hard to maintain his equanimity, and the father found more excuses to delay payment. Eventually the treatment stopped with the therapist owed a vast sum, the girl being far from ready to end, and the father confirmed in his omnipotent belief that he could destroy any male rival.

If these administrative issues are not realistically addressed in a way that is consistent with forging an open and collaborative therapeutic alliance with patients, the treatment may eventually founder. In line with the idea of a collaborative relationship and open-system rootedness in reality, we give adult patients, parents, and child and adolescent patients clear statements and explanations of our working arrangements at the stage of making the recommendation for treatment. There is a chance to talk these through and address questions and issues at the outset so that no one is surprised.

What Are the Working Arrangements?

Each therapist develops their own practices, but we have found that it establishes a backstop against which resistances and conflicts may be measured if we start with explicit guidelines. Most important is that the evaluation establishes the idea that everything has meaning; then our working arrangements are not seen only as idiosyncratic whims but as ways of conveying and establishing the importance of the treatment to all parties. We explain and discuss our fees, billing practices, responsibility for missed sessions, illnesses, vacations, rescheduling, modes of communication, and so forth. We ask for payment to be made at the same regular time each month.

Are Some Working Arrangements More Important than Others?

All the working arrangements have impact and each of them will probably be co-opted by patients into the service of defensive needs or aggressive wishes at some point in the treatment. To safeguard the treatment from premature termination and allow time for addressing such issues, we have found it crucial to establish that no changes will be made in the treatment arrangements by the patient, parents, or therapist without thirty days' notice.

All therapists have experienced painful summary withdrawals, premature terminations, or unilateral announcements of reductions in the frequency of sessions, and so forth. By setting up a mutually agreed policy to ensure thirty days to work together before any change, we have found that many treatments can be saved. This is particularly important in work with adolescents, who often use attendance as an expression of conflict. With time to work on the issues, as well as the incentive that the sessions will have to be paid for anyway, most patients engage in the work of examining the problem. The idea of thirty days' notice concretizes the seriousness of the mutual commitment patients and therapists are making.

> A young adult who was struggling in his work setting, feeling that everyone hated him and was out to get him, sought treatment. He accepted the recommendation for therapy but soon brought his paranoid thinking into the treatment and, by the second session, gave thirty days' notice of stopping. He continued to do this monthly for the next two years, each time ostensibly around a different issue. The agreed provision of thirty days' notice allowed for working on his extreme anxiety about commitment and emotional involvement, and he was eventually able to move into a period of fruitful therapeutic work and then have a planned termination period.[7]

What Are the Positive and Negative Possibilities for Termination at the Evaluation Phase?

Each phase of treatment contains the potential for movement in the direction of a planned, genuine, growth-enhancing termination. Equally, each phase has particular pitfalls in relation to termination, which can lead to a premature ending.

At the evaluation phase, a refusal to accept the recommendation for treatment may represent a unilateral termination. It is our impression, which is borne out by research on populations of all ages, that large numbers of patients refuse treatment recommendations.[8] By taking note of the patient's history of leave-taking and linking the past to current anxiety, therapists may forestall refusal of treatment.

On the positive side, the evaluation includes beginning a wide range of transformations. Details of the transformations initiated first in the evaluation/exploratory phase can be found in the Therapeutic Alliance Table at the back of the book. These set the stage for eventual consolidation of open-system functioning through the mourning that recurs in increments throughout treatment and promotes the adaptive internalization that is part of a mutually agreed-upon termination.

Notes

1 Sroufe 2021

2 Ferraro and Garella (2009) credit our contribution of this link between adolescence and premature termination as central to their model.

3 Ferenczi and Rank 1924.

4 Goin, Yamamoto, and Silverman 1965.

5 J. Novick and K.K. Novick 2000.

6 K.K. Novick and J. Novick 2005, 2013, 2020, 2022.

7 In the 32 cases collected in the Parent Work Casebook (Editors K.K. Novick et al 2021) and the Adolescent Casebook (Editors J. Novick and K.K. Novick 2022) there was a pervasive finding that premature terminations related to either too short an evaluation or a lack of a contract for sufficient notice of changes in treatment frame.

8 Novick, Benson and Rembar 1981.

3

Beginning Phase

What Can You See at the Beginning Phase of Treatment That Is Relevant to Termination?

During the beginning phase, we focus on the conditions the patient sets up for *being with* the therapist. Regarding termination, we look particularly at what the patient does to feel safe and in control in relation to *separations*. In recent years, authors such as Bergmann,[1] Craige,[2] Pinsky,[3] and others have commented that therapy involves an ending that has no precedent or analogue in ordinary life experience. Many patients sense this during the evaluation, as they are helped to find courage to commit to a treatment that requires a positive attachment but also has a built-in ending. In the beginning phase, both partners in the journey are getting to know each other, and both have the knowledge that this relationship will end.

Long before you can address deep separation themes, you can see the patient's reactions to separation on weekends, holidays, and vacations. This will become important knowledge for dealing with the pretermination and termination phases. Simultaneously, therapists can monitor their own reactions to separation and sort out open- and closed-system attachments to the patient.[4]

What Are the Different Reactions to Separation You Can See at the Beginning Phase?

1. Denial: the patient may act as if a weekend or vacation break did not happen

2. Denial of significance of a past or upcoming break, with or without anger

3. Opposite reaction: desperate clinging and dependency

4. Intellectualized acknowledgment that it matters

5. Acting out, for instance, the patient unexpectedly canceling sessions before or after the therapist's absence

6. Conscious withholding of thoughts and feelings

7. Genuine working with thoughts, feelings, and reactions

How Can You Address Denial?

Keeping termination issues in mind, even at the beginning of treatment, helps us to be appropriately active, for instance, taking the initiative to remark on patterns of reactions to separations:

"Have you noticed that you have not mentioned . . .?"

"Sometimes things that are omitted turn out to be important: you haven't mentioned the recent break."

Interventions such as these are directed to helping patients learn to observe themselves, a component of the self-reflective function usually considered an important criterion for termination.

How Can You Address Denial of the Significance of the Break?

This presents an opportunity to demystify treatment and enlist the patient in a joint endeavor. We can say, for instance, "Here we can look at and work on issues that many avoid throughout life—hellos and goodbyes. We can look at the solutions you find to deal with such moments. Avoidance is one solution, not to have feelings."

Or we can offer treatment as an opportunity to open things up and explore or play with them in a miniature, safe setting, that is, when it is a weekend, not a death. This allows for seeing what the dimensions of the issue are. It is rather like going to a play that depicts strong events and emotions; you feel them intensely but in a time-limited way.

Working on the defensive pattern of denying the emotional significance of a separation helps us prepare for the patient's later pattern of termination. The patient's capacity to acknowledge feelings is the first step in the long journey toward open-system self-regulation of emotions, which becomes a criterion for starting a pretermination phase.

If the patient gets angry about these interventions, we can suggest that we look together at why these questions generate so much heat. This avenue of inquiry will open up issues of helplessness, anger, control, guilt, and omnipotent ideas, which all pertain to closed-system solutions. A major issue for pretermination is whether the patient is able to set aside related omnipotent beliefs.

This kind of denial often reveals a belief that having feelings about the therapist is a sign of weakness that threatens self-esteem or aspects of identity, including gender identity.

Larry came from a long line of military men and had been brought up to be a "brave soldier" who never cried. He was insulted when I wondered about his feelings around weekends and vacations. I pointed out that hellos and goodbyes are universally meaningful experiences and that a persistent pattern of no reaction is as significant as an overt reaction. Describing these times as opportunities to look at his feelings and understand their significance instead of ignoring them helped bring Larry's family history of stoicism and its meaning in his relationship with his father into the treatment. Moving beyond his father was eventually a critical issue in Larry's termination.

Mrs. T kept herself in the beginning phase of treatment for a long time by denying any emotions around separation in her life or analysis. Thus I had ample notice that this would be a long and arduous treatment, with changes coming slowly and only after painstaking and piecemeal advances. For me it was important to hold on to the framework of termination dimensions throughout treatment, in order to assess the full significance of Mrs. T's denial. This could be understood as Mrs. T's implementation of her lifelong pattern of refusing to take the initiative; if she had feelings, she would have to act. She feared risking desire or action and used a passive, helpless stance to force the other person always to be in charge. We will return to Mrs. T's dilemma in discussing middle-phase conflicts over creativity that threatened to bring her analysis to a standstill and halt progress toward termination.

Looking at reactions to ordinary separations can alert us to the scale of defenses against any positive feelings, especially love. Such patients may be very young children diagnosed as autistic or adolescents who present as severely obsesssive-compulsive or psychopathic—we have to consider the threats to experiencing an ordinary full range of emotions that have impacted the individual patient in the course of development.[5] We listen for patterns of self-protection in reaction to trauma, neglect, abuse, or repeated experiences of rejection, exclusion, prejudice, and discrimination.

How Can You Deal with Clinging, Dependency, and Rage about Separation?

These feelings are not restricted to termination issues, but extreme separation reactions at the beginning of treatment signal that they may be difficult throughout.

Mrs. C, a successful and capable professional, sought treatment to deal with her depression and rage. Very soon after starting therapy, she reacted to weekends and vacations intensely. She felt panicky and needed to know where I would be and arranged to telephone at regular times during my vacation. Work on the early determinants of her fear that I might die during the absence helped to allay some of her terror, but it was clear to both of us that separation would remain a central issue and would affect Mrs. C's capacity to move toward termination.

Miss D, a college student, also had extreme reactions to separation. Every time I was away for more than a few days, she had multiple accidents, stepping out in front of cars, crashing her bicycle into lampposts, burning herself on the stove in her apartment. This was alarming to me, as Miss D affected not to realize the pattern until it had repeated multiple times. Eventually we were able to understand together that Miss D was externalizing her own capacity to be a good internal parent to herself onto me, in hopes that I would take over and keep her safe. Simultaneously, as a function of her history of abuse, she needed to keep proving that I could not keep her any safer than her assaultive, incompetent mother had. Her prevalent use of externalization alerted me to an important dynamic that would affect termination later.

Externalization is a major defense mechanism used for the maintenance of sadomasochistic relationships. It is abusive in itself, as it denies the reality and individuality of the other person, imposing characteristics and aspects of the self that the patient finds unbearable to own.[6] As long as patients use externalization as a major component of their defensive repertoire, they will be unable to move forward toward termination, since a genuine good-bye involves mourning, the recognition that there is a valued, loved, real other whom the person is sad to leave.

Mastery of feelings is an important goal in relation to pretermination and termination, and patients who have trouble modulating their emotions have a sizable task ahead. Their treatments will probably be long. The danger of an interminable treatment arises here, or the therapist's reaction may lead to a forced termination. This would represent an enactment of rejection, in which the therapist becomes the aggressor. Early indicators can appear in the therapist's acting out by being late, forgetting the patient, mistaking times, and so on. Often, these are patients who anticipate rejection, provoke rejection from others, and will attempt to do so with the therapist as well.

Mrs. N, a divorced middle-aged mother of two grown children, had been in various forms of therapy since a suicide attempt in high school. She had nothing but criticism and complaints about each of her therapists, her former husband, and a series of men who had disappointed her or betrayed her trust. She started her treatment with great hopes and nothing but praise for my therapeutic skills. The first long weekend happened a few months after the start of treatment, and she spoke of how hard she found the separation; she said that she could not imagine how she would deal with the longer planned vacations or the eventual end of treatment. Soon after, she began telephoning on weekends, often at inconvenient times. She did not seem to benefit from these calls or respond to work on the meaning or purpose of these intrusions. She believed that she could counter helplessness by controlling our interactions in this way. I became frustrated and was tempted to not pick up the phone when I saw her name on the caller ID. We then talked about how it is almost always possible to evoke negative feelings in others, and then she could feel in control. It took much further work for us to arrive at her fear of helplessness to guarantee my positive responses and find alternative ways of interacting that she could begin to trust.

Are There Other Termination Dangers in the Beginning Phase?

In child and adolescent treatment, loyalty conflicts can quickly arise. If they go unrecognized and if children and parents are not helped to deal with them, parents are likely to pull the child out of treatment.

Adolescents cling to their externalizing defenses, and the analyst and the treatment can be experienced as threatening the tenuous equilibrium the adolescent has set up. To avoid a precipitate flight from treatment, we try to find the progressive, adaptive component in the externalized solution. For instance, the patient's blaming of parents can include also a wish to be independent; promiscuity can represent a distorted expression of the wish to own the body; drug use can include a yearning for independence, acceptance, and good feelings.

A sixteen-year-old boy was brought for treatment because his frantic parents couldn't understand why his grades had plummeted and he had become uncommunicative and unmotivated. Earl reluctantly participated in the evaluation and grudgingly accepted treatment, largely to get his parents off his back but also curious about my interest in his mind-expanding reaction to a variety of drugs, including LSD. Earl was using drugs to deal with severe social anxiety and fear of girls. But with the drugs he wasn't actually experiencing the anxiety, thus obviating a potential motivation for therapy. He challenged me, saying, "I have no problems except my parents, and I'm here because my parents have made me come, but I'm not sticking around." I verbalized Earl's excitement about his creative ideas in his LSD experiences and suggested that it would be interesting to find out if he could access these feelings without the drugs and then put the ideas into action. The excitement Earl felt on drugs was about his creative capacity that he inhibited ordinarily. Once I explicitly shared Earl's creative joy and sympathized with the painful frustration Earl went through when this was stymied by his inhibitions, Earl could feel that there was something to work on in treatment and resolved to stay.

Parents may be threatened by their fears that the therapist will be a rival or a better parent. To deal with this fear, they may try to get the therapist to collude with them as an enforcer of their moral or social strictures. If we do not handle this with tact, an adolescent patient will see us as an agent of the parents and bolt. Refusal to join the parents, however, produces a reaction in them. Parents may then see us as foolish, seductive, or incompetent and pull the adolescent out of treatment. Adolescent patients are adept at splitting and manipulating these situations; hence the high proportion of premature terminations of adolescent treatments and the importance of addressing these issues to maintain the work and avoid interruptions.[7]

Neglecting to notice and reinforce positive parental feelings causes many therapeutic failures early in the treatment of young people. One contributor to such a failure is the prevalent pattern of treating late adolescents as adults, with no explicit provision for the specific needs of parents and young people during this phase of development, as they become late adolescents and emerging adults. We have defined the parents' therapeutic alliance task at the beginning of treatment as allowing the child to make a significant relationship with another adult. We can devise techniques that both protect the patient's working toward being with the therapist and address parental anxieties and conflicts over allowing the therapeutic relationship to develop.

Part of the discussion of the working arrangements during the evaluation involves planning with the patient for meeting the parents' needs in relation to the treatment. Our general model includes regular dynamic concurrent parent work throughout the young person's treatment to address the progressive transformation of the parent-child relationship from both sides. Occasional formal joint sessions may be useful in some situations. We have found it helpful to say explicitly that therapy with children and adolescents has dual goals: restoration of the patient to the path of progressive development and transformation of the parent-child relationship to a lifelong resource for both.[8]

The importance of including parents in the ongoing work is exemplified in the contrast between two adolescents: an eighteen-year-old in treatment with no ancillary parent work and a nineteen-year-old with parent work done consistently from the start of treatment at sixteen.

In the first case, treatment started when the boy was seventeen because of school failure. His parents were seen only briefly during the evaluation. Jeremy made considerable improvement in the first months of work: he was less depressed, his grades improved, and he was feeling better about himself. He had been smoking marijuana since middle school, and, at times, he seriously abused the drug, staying stoned for days on end. One day he was caught at school with marijuana in his car and was suspended. His father was in a rage. Both parents felt that treatment had been a failure and peremptorily ended his therapy.

Janet also presented with serious school problems, depression, and self-destructive behavior. She too made significant progress, but when she started college, she began to abuse alcohol, sometimes becoming "wasted" to the point that she could not remember the events the following day. We were addressing this issue when Janet wrecked her car while driving drunk. She was fortunate that no one was seriously hurt. Her mother was furious and wanted to punish Janet to "teach her responsibility."

I had met regularly with Janet's mother and stepfather during the high school years and continued to do so when Janet started college. The mother called me and expressed her rage and frustration, saying how much she wanted to punish Janet but said, "I wanted to talk to you first." A series of meetings with Janet and her parents led to working out a reparative program that everyone could feel comfortable with. Most importantly, it maintained the loving, supportive tie between parents and child, which had been worked on earlier. Janet's treatment resumed, and important inroads were made on Janet's self-destructive rage when she had been left by a boyfriend and the roots of this reaction in her early abandonment by her father.

With adults, if the evaluation has begun the transformation of distorted fantasies and expectations about treatment, there are two main termination-related dangers in the beginning phase.

The Impact of Pathological Closed-System Patterns in the Patient's Ongoing Relationships

When we apply lessons from adolescent work, we may see how profoundly therapy will disrupt established patterns of relationships in the patient's life. A loyalty conflict may be set up in the patient, where, for example, the significant other may feel threatened or, alternatively, seek to bring the therapist into a compact to force changes on the patient.

Mr. D, a successful entrepreneur, was pushed into treatment by his wife, who threatened divorce if he did not deal with his addiction to internet pornography. Even though he was a highly accomplished middle-aged man with three teenaged children, he came to treatment like a sulky adolescent, for whom treatment was a punishment rather than a personal opportunity for growth. His plan was clearly to leave as soon as possible.

Rather than following his wife's agenda, Mr. D and I sought to discover what legitimate need he was trying to meet with his internet addiction. Only when watching porn did he feel in charge of his activities, rather than being totally controlled by his very disturbed wife. What emerged were his legitimate wishes for psychological autonomy. On this basis, he was motivated to continue treatment to seek more adaptive ways to meet that need.

Both People Settling into an Empathic Bog

The second danger is an interminable beginning phase, in which a treatment never moves beyond the initial phase of being with and feeling with. The patient is only seen as traumatized, dependent, and needing reparative love. The therapist is cast in and revels in the role of the perfect mother/parent who, through the power of love and sacrifice, can cure all. In this scenario, patients can never proceed to a good ending until the treatment moves beyond the first understanding, however authentic, of their being only the passive victim of traumatic events to their active use of the victim stance to enforce their will on others. When we begin to see the maintenance of the passive, victimized position as the closed-system solution the patient has arrived at to feel connected, safe, and gratified, we can communicate the understanding that this was a powerful, effective solution to the patient's experience of helplessness at the time. The cost, however, was very high, and so it will be worth working in therapy to find alternative means to protect the self.

In a different scenario, the roles can be reversed, and the therapist can be the helpless, bewildered one, while the patient controls the interaction through hostile externalizations of inadequacies. These are the treatments that end prematurely or persist for years fruitlessly, leaving both people unsatisfied. Schlesinger pointed out that, in interminable treatments, "What therapist and patient are doing has ceased to be psychotherapy some time ago when it metamorphosed into a relationship that constitutes its own reward, perhaps for both parties."[9] There are many published examples of interminable treatments that fit Schlesinger's description, notably many of the cases in Salberg's edited collection on termination from a relational perspective.[10]

At some point, we may introduce the idea of "emotional muscle," the capacity to tolerate and master affects. With parental support, children learn to deal with the ordinary frustrations and obstacles of life and develop the emotional muscle to handle ordinary levels of psychic discomfort. The good-enough parent does not, and in fact cannot, remove all obstacles, anticipate all frustrations and conflicts, and protect her child from all uncomfortable feelings. The attempt to do so undermines the growth of the child's emotional strength. Emotional muscle can turn a state of rage into a signal affect; building emotional muscle leads to resiliency, the quality that differentiates outcomes to trauma.

By keeping in mind the idea of treatment progression and movement through the phases in the direction of a mutually satisfying and constructive ending, we increase our awareness of the defenses and relationship patterns that can undermine the potential for a good goodbye. Knowledge of the goals and prerequisites for a good ending helps us generate techniques to master and move beyond a sadomasochistic transference in the beginning phase.

How Is the Transition from the Beginning Phase of Treatment to the Middle Phase Marked?

There are many indicators of this important shift:

1. There is an increased capacity to regulate intense feelings, modulating emotional states into signal affect, which is a beginning development of "emotional muscle."
2. There is an increased focus on how the patient's mind works.
3. Patients seem more curious about themselves.
4. Patients show improved ability for self-observation.

The next three markers are particularly relevant to a good ending, as they represent open-system dimensions of the treatment experience, which the patient will internalize for post-termination living:

5. There is a significant increase in the joint activity and endeavor of patient and therapist working together. There is greater shared curiosity and wish to understand fluctuations in working together as they arise from different sources. The fluctuations are experienced as interferences in thinking and in thinking together and can be tracked by both people.

6. The patient shows an increased capacity to play.

7. The patient takes more pleasure in the process and the experience of working together and alone.

How Does This Transition Relate to Termination?

Work on reactions to separation has created conditions of greater security and object constancy. This creates a space for collaboration and strengthens the realistic interdependence of patient and therapist. These elements are crucial to determining the timing of termination.

Separation issues are important in any treatment but take on particular significance through the lens of termination, since termination of therapy is separation from a person with whom the patient has shared a very intense and meaningful relationship. Patients will have both real and fantasy attachments to us, all of which have to be understood together. The fantasies about the self and the other will eventually have to be set aside, whereas the realities can be internalized and identified with in the service of growth. All this holds for the therapist as well.

Schlesinger noted that every resolution of a conflict is an achievement but also represents the loss of an earlier solution. This duality reminds us of the resonances of termination present in the movement through all phases of treatment. The repetition of achievement and loss throughout treatment strengthens the emotional muscles needed to bear sadness, mourn, and grow from termination.

Mr. N often made me feel ineffectual. He said he couldn't bear to lie on the couch or sit in a chair facing me and ended up sitting behind me, so that I couldn't see him. I sought consultation around my own feelings of confusion, as well as my anger at feeling forced to do something I didn't usually do. I considered ideas about externalization and childhood abuse, but these were of little use to me at that point. I then decided to relax and let it be. If that was the only way he could be with me and it didn't represent a danger to anyone, then I shouldn't interfere but experience it together with him, "feel with" him, and work to understand his needs with him.

Toward the end of the lengthy beginning phase of his treatment, he said, "I really look forward to coming here. This is the only place I can tell someone the wacky things that go on in my head. But when I get here, I choke up, and I just can't say what I want to say." Mr. N had moved into a treatment relationship in which he could find a way to be with me and begin to experience the conflict between his wish to share his thoughts and the powerful anxieties that stopped him. This indicated his transition into the middle phase of working together, and this progression presaged his eventual capacity to have a good ending.

Notes

1 Bergmann 1988.

2 Craige 2002, 2009.

3 Pinsky 2002.

4 See J. Novick and K. K. Novick (2000), "Love in the Therapeutic Alliance," for a detailed exploration of open- and closed-system love and the role of the therapist's feelings in termination.

5 See the work of Singletary (2023) on difficulties in receiving love or help, and Aichorn on work with delinquent youth ([1935] 1984).

6 J. Novick and K.K. Novick 1994.

7 K.K. Novick and J. Novick 2005.

8 K.K. Novick and J. Novick 2005, 2013, 2020; J. Novick and K.K. Novick 2022.

9 Schlesinger [2005] 2013, p. 50.

10 Salberg 2010.

4

Middle Phase

What Characterizes the Middle Phase of Treatment in Relation to Termination?

The relatively long middle phase of therapy is when the therapist and patient address issues about the patient's mind—how it works and how it joins with other minds, particularly the therapist's, in working together toward a goal.

In relation to termination, the work of the middle phase facilitates the increasing emergence of open-system functioning, so that the patient can experience an internal conflict between the two systems of self-regulation. Over time, closed-system functioning has become an addiction (both psychologically and physiologically), and we know that a person can only begin to control addiction when good alternatives are available. Experience of this conflict provides patients with a genuine choice, the incentive to set aside closed-system solutions and gratifications and discover, even if fleetingly at first, that the open system offers more dependable and genuine pleasures at lower cost. This is a crucial part of progression toward termination. At the same time, this conflict intensifies anxiety about an eventual end and manifests increasingly in the therapeutic relationship.

How Does Internal Conflict between the Two Systems Manifest Itself during the Middle Phase?

Conflict between the two systems shows in the areas of relationships, work, and feelings. These are not mutually exclusive arenas, but it is clearer to describe them separately.

What Is the Conflict in the Area of Relationships?

Adults experience a conflict between two different ways of relating to the self and to others. Objective love for the therapist develops in the middle phase, and this threatens old, pathological, transference ways of relating based on omnipotent delusions of forcing and controlling others.[1] Love of the process is achieved and lost, then regained; these fluctuations allow for contrasting perceptions of different ways of experiencing good feelings with others. Competing sources of self-esteem are increasingly evident.

> I tracked Mr. G's good feelings in the sessions, noting when he enjoyed coming, used his mind, and felt good about having his normal ego needs met: to be listened to, understood, and respected. Mr. G recaptured early memories of his grandmother, who had loved him and treated him as a worthy individual. This recovery of a loving, joyful aspect of himself constituted the other side of the conflict with an omnipotent, magical, destructive self. The omnipotent defenses made him feel strong and powerful; his love brought joy but left him feeling vulnerable, especially to abandonment. Focus on his feelings about being with me and working with me allowed for a full experience of his conflict between two ways of functioning. There was a gradual expansion of pleasure from competence in his external life, particularly at work, where his organizational and research activities became noticeably more successful and his interactions with colleagues improved. Mr. G attributed this shift to the therapy and was very appreciative.
>
> However, Mr. G maintained and protected closed-system functioning in his relationship with his wife, whom he bullied and yelled at on weekends.

He forced her to submit physically and sexually to his demands. Through his grandmother transference to me, he had recovered an open-system way of relating. I could see the conflict and mutually exclusive nature of these two ways of relating, but Mr. G clung to the omnipotent idea that he could have both.

How Can the Therapist Help?

In other writings, we have noted that sadomasochistic omnipotent beliefs are elements in all pathologies, cutting across diagnostic categories. We have emphasized the closed-system solutions as a defense that most patients will do anything to protect, including self-injury or suicide.[2] Without the open competent system as a viable alternative, patients have little incentive to change the adaptations they have clung to, perhaps from earliest childhood. Patients usually come for help because their omnipotent solutions are not working well enough. They then press to cast the therapist as another omnipotent figure they can control by sadomasochistic means.

Genuinely nonexploitative joint work threatens a stable sadomasochistic character organization that seeks to turn treatment into a never-ending perverse gratification. Sadomasochism has determinants from all levels of development, serves multiple functions, and is a very difficult pathology to deal with. Hostile omnipotent beliefs form a triumphant, self-protective shell in power relationships, and patients may go to extreme lengths rather than relinquish them.

> Mr. G's awareness of an alternative, even though he was not yet committed to it, nor able to function in an open-system way with his wife, was a major step in his progression. I was encouraged by being able to imagine a pathway to a good goodbye.

What Is the Conflict in the Area of Work?

Middle-phase therapeutic effort leads eventually to the patient experiencing competing sources of satisfaction. One is the old quick, easy, closed-system, magical omnipotent solution where wishing will make it so. Cheating, plagiarism, delinquency and idleness avoid the necessity to work to solve problems, in or out of treatment. This familiar gratification is hard to set aside. In contrast, increasing experiences of joy and pleasure in creativity and competence begin to shift the balance. Open-system functioning with its real impacts and authentic satisfactions starts to feel possible. These fluctuating experiences can be painful and demanding. The achievements of the middle phase are crucial building blocks of the restructured personality that will be ready for a good ending, but they can revive old fears and conflicts about the meaning of change and growth. They also evoke old defensive responses to such feelings. Schlesinger too described this arduous oscillation as change begins to take hold.[3]

> With continued attention to Mrs. T's externalizations of ego functions, she gradually became more involved in the analytic work, marking her transition into the middle phase of treatment. But this led to memories of failure and overwhelming feelings of humiliation. Interpretation of the link to her experiences with a mother who used shame and invidious comparison with a preferred older brother only intensified her reluctance to take the initiative. At times it was painfully difficult for Mrs. T to reflect, expand, associate, or explore her ego functioning. The source of the humiliation was by that time lodged in her own ego ideal, her own demand that she be always right, that she be perfect or go away and practice in secret until she achieved perfection: "I will not tolerate mediocrity in myself. I have to be perfect or work on it until I am." All positive, supportive comments made her feel like a helpless, defective child. She was in the throes of a full-blown sadomasochistic transference neurosis and threatened to leave treatment.[4] Open-system working together is incompatible with sadomasochism. This was a serious therapeutic crisis, but Mrs. T and I found a way out through her stories.

How Can the Therapist Help?

In the course of treatment, Mrs. T had developed an interest in writing stories, enrolled in a number of writing classes, and then began sharing the stories in her sessions, sometimes reading drafts or sections to me. At no time did she expect or ask for a literary critique but explicitly used the stories to explore the inner lives of her characters. For quite a while I made no link between a particular character and the patient, but sometimes, in relation to a particular facet of a character's described personality, Mrs. T would say, "That's like me."

This continued for some time, as the stories changed and a few were published. I was occasionally concerned that treatment had turned into a literary seminar. Despite moments of doubt, I generally trusted a feeling of momentum generated by the joint attention made possible by the focus on fictional characters. We were working together, even if the focus was not always obviously on Mrs. T.

I made a technical choice not to interpret the closed-system defensiveness but to support open-system elements. With space to work together on understanding the stories, Mrs. T discovered a potential source of self-esteem in feelings of competence and efficacy from the work, rather than from controlling me. She began to track patterns of fluent thinking, constrictions, and fuzziness, which were noted, then altered and mastered. From a developmental perspective, this part of the treatment resembled child work, where a play space is established that allows for talking about and working on conflicts first in displacement, as in doll play or games. For the first time, I felt secure about the stability and progression of the treatment. Unilateral termination seemed less imminent, and the increase in open-system functioning made the prospect of a good ending imaginable.

Working together, whether in the patient's life at work and home or in the treatment, is a mixed experience that brings great satisfaction in the process and achievement of understanding and includes inevitable disappointments at limitations in insight, difficulties in communication, and transient dyssynchronies between patient and analyst. This workaday task of the therapeutic alliance brings out the delusional image of a perfect communion that many patients strive for but also allows for the repair of the mismatch, which is a crucial component of early developmental experience.[5] The therapeutic alliance issues highlight the transference reenactment of problematic relationships with past and present people in the patient's life and their conflicts over wishing for perfection, as well as pointing the way toward different solutions in different ways of relating.

What Is the Conflict in the Area of Feelings?

Working together effectively provides intense satisfaction that draws first on the accumulated transformations of early experiences of attunement. Second, working well provides a shared experience of actual competence that stands in contrast to a closed system of pleasure from magical beliefs of omnipotent control over others. Reality-oriented satisfaction motivates further collaborative work. The pleasure of accomplishing the middle-phase task of working together leads to the internalization of dialogue and exploration and nourishes creativity, with its accompanying feelings of joy. Repeated experience of pleasure from competence is necessary for the patient to develop a conflict between different ways of regulating self-esteem. One of the goals of the middle phase is to help the patient experience an alternative in the emotions associated with the open, competent system of self-regulation. These encompass attachment through objective love, rather than fantasies of control by enthrallment or submission, and the use of feelings such as anger, anxiety, or excitement as signals for reality engagement rather than means to overwhelm and force another person.

> Another patient, Ms. H, had reacted intensely during the evaluation to even my minor interventions and found it almost impossible to take anything in when she began to feel too much. Through the beginning of treatment, Ms. H talked a lot, jumping from subject to subject. Sometimes she told me not to speak because she could not listen. The threat of her extreme emotions began to create a controlling atmosphere. I was alternately annoyed and worried about whether the patient was more disturbed than she had appeared.
>
> Ms. H's extreme need to control created a barrier to progress and a pressure for a relationship ruled by intense, full-blown affects. From the beginning I frequently described her tendency to flood us both with her feelings as evidencing her belief in the omnipotent power of feelings. I then contrasted this with the idea of using feelings as signals to help mobilize

her keen problem-solving abilities. She had never thought of feelings as useful signals and didn't believe she could do this. Focusing consistently on the strengths of her personality helped Ms. H respond to the steadiness of my regard with a gradual expansion of her emotional range and repertoire. She responded positively to the idea, so useful in child and applied work, of developing "emotional muscle," that is, increasing flexibility and resilience in tolerating emotions.[6] She found new ways to be with me and participate in the work of the treatment, which augured well for her growing capacity to tolerate the feelings eventually associated with termination.

How Great Is the Danger of Premature Termination in the Middle Phase of Treatment?

The middle phase brings a high risk of premature termination, second only to the time of making the recommendation for treatment, at which point so many patients balk. The work of the middle phase has brought the open system into play. In contrast to the timeless, unrealistic universe of the closed system, the open system is rooted in the reality of change. This is a manifestation of what has been called the "growth principle," the idea that development is intrinsic to mental life.[7] Issues of change, progression, loss, sadness, and mortality are inevitably present. The pull to closed-system denial of the realities of gender, generation, and time is intense. Resistances can take many forms, from conscious refusal to think about the future to unconscious maintenance of pathological patterns or precipitating a unilateral premature termination.

What Is Going On in the Patient Who Denies Change?

Some patients deny the evident changes, holding on to their closed-system solutions and consciously withholding information about gains outside therapy. This dynamic has a direct bearing on termination, as exploration often reveals that the patient is afraid that the gains inevitably imply ending the treatment. Another possibility is attributing the changes to anything but the therapy, citing the season, a new job, or the advice of a friend. Along with benefits that may accrue from psychotropic medications, there is a potential for misuse. Many patients seek medication at this point in their treatment in order to be able to deny the impact of the therapeutic relationship and the work that is going on. There is genuine pain associated with setting aside both the real and the illusory gains of familiar closed-system functioning; this can lead to acute conflicts in the middle phase.

Others deny change in a more complex way: this can take the form of complaining about the therapy and looking for other modalities of treatment, thought to be miraculously more effective or tailored to fantasy ideals. This is often the repetition of an adolescent pattern of leave-taking, which was used at that time to avoid sadness and mourning.

What Does It Mean When the Patient Makes Staying in Treatment the Therapist's Issue?

Some patients may angrily reject the therapist with the accusation that the therapist is "clinging" when the therapist suggests the need for continued work. First, it is important for the therapist to check whether they are indeed holding on to the patient in an obstructive way, not respecting the patient's newfound capacities. If they are not, however, then the patient may be conflating autonomy and separation. A person can be autonomous without leaving. Indeed, in the course of development, autonomy should come well before significant separation. A person can also separate without being autonomous, which often occurs at adolescence when a youngster is prematurely expected to leave home.[8]

Seventeen-year-old Daniel's analysis had been proceeding well, with marked improvement in his social and academic functioning. His father was anxious for him to finish treatment, as he "seemed completely cured." In the treatment, Daniel was experiencing anxiety about what finishing would mean. As he talked about these fears, he first expressed his wish to leave, and then he became anxious. Soon, however, this turned to defensive bravado, and he scornfully gave me a tissue, saying that I shouldn't "cry like a snot-nosed ten-year-old."

At this point I remembered the beginning of Daniel's treatment, when Daniel had described himself as a "snot-nosed ten-year-old" at the time of his mother's death. Daniel was externalizing the helpless, abandoned little boy aspect of himself onto me and planned to leave it behind. Rather than a process of leave-taking between differentiated, whole, real people in the present, Daniel was attempting an omnipotent unilateral solution to his anxieties about the future.

Is This Related to Dependency Issues? How Does It Connect to Termination?

Patients with intense conflicts around dependency needs often announce this at the beginning of treatment or even in the evaluation. "There's no way I am going to stay here forever." Or, "I will certainly never have a transference to you." These difficulties play a large part during the beginning phase of treatment, and they recur in the middle phase in relation to good feelings from working together. Patients may get anxious that they will never want to leave. The fear is that the love will make them lose themselves. A major source of danger is anxiety and conflict around pleasure in working together and love for the person with whom one does that. Then the risk is of a premature leaving fueled by a need to destroy love in the service of preserving a false idea of autonomy.

How Can the Therapist Address the Fear of Love and Pleasure?

With some patients, the conflict over allowing themselves to feel pleasure and to risk good feelings with another person is evident from the evaluation, as we saw in chapter 2. For others, the difficulty in feeling, holding on to, and trusting pleasure, satisfaction, and mastery emerges gradually with the help of the therapist in pointing out repeated instances. The related thread of loving feelings is a pervasive theme, underground for some, more visible in others, that therapists address throughout the phases of treatment.

By the middle phase, with its satisfying experience of shared and collaborative exercise of both minds, we can see that the patient's capacity for objective love of self and others is expanding, as is the therapist's appreciation for this person's unique self. We can address fluctuations in trust in loving feelings and explore together what gets in the way of and what fosters restoration of the patient's capacity for love in general. As these issues are canvassed, we can bring them into the context of eventual termination, when love for the therapist can be spread to other relationships.

What Are Other Issues in the Middle Phase that Might Lead to Premature Termination?

Parents often pull children and adolescents out of treatment because they feel threatened by the child's eagerness and pleasure in the work and the relationship. The child or adolescent has developed love with content, based on shared experience of mastery and ongoing work. When parents realize that this is not just a honeymoon, as it can be at the beginning of treatment, their own self-esteem and defenses can be assailed.

With adults, as we saw in the cases described above, the conscious experience of conflict between open- and closed-system ways of functioning puts pressure on the treatment. The satisfaction, creative joy, and objective love for the self and the other threaten old closed-system patterns of defense against helplessness, trauma, anxiety, and depression. In many cases, however, patients fight awareness of this conflict. Then a pattern similar to the one we see in child and adolescent work may ensue, in which the spouse or significant other is unconsciously enlisted in the service of sabotaging the treatment or even ending it prematurely.

We strongly advise dynamic concurrent parent work throughout a child's or adolescent's treatment, whenever possible, in order to restore the parent-child relationship to primary love and strength. Parents are in the midst of their own developmental process that can be supported and nurtured by regular attention to the parenting function; the dynamic changes in their child promote changes in parents. When we stay aware of responses in an adult patient's significant others to the treatment, the therapist, and the changes that are ongoing, we can then examine with the patient what they are communicating or not, and how they are or are not working with their significant other to grow together. When the therapist keeps these dimensions in mind throughout, we reduce the risk of abrupt terminations.

What If There Are External Reasons for Ending?

Often patients bring external reasons for ending rather than internal readiness. This may be a job in another city, a family obligation, pressure from spouse or parent, and so forth. The therapist is initially put in a position that is potentially adversarial and can lead back to a closed-system interaction. The patient will either overpower the therapist or submit. Either way, they are reverting to sadomasochistic relating. The therapist has the task of holding back from being pulled into such an interaction and then reminding the patient of the goals they had set together, with a view to looking together at where they are in relation to those goals.

After some time in treatment, there had been significant improvement in many areas of Mrs. F's functioning. She announced one day that her husband had taken a position in another city and she would have to go with him. I wondered why she felt she "had" to go and if this way of leaving me and her therapeutic work might be a repetition of an old pattern. She then elaborated on something she had previously touched on only briefly. She said that her first year of college had been at an exciting, stimulating Eastern university, but her father had decided that she should transfer to a small, Southern religious school thereafter. The patient had docilely accepted this decision. When I suggested a possible link between the excitement of her first year at college and her feelings about her treatment, Mrs. F could see that her passive compliance with her husband's move paralleled her willingness to accept her father's decision. In both instances, under the guise of a helpless submissiveness, there was an active attempt to avoid not only possible transference fantasies but also open-system growth and accompanying pleasure and autonomy. She came to feel that she had been "running for long enough" and that it was time to turn around and face these issues. She worked out with her husband that she would not move right away but would stay until her treatment had reached a satisfactory stopping point.

Such dynamic issues are important to keep in mind when faced with external realities such as those brought by Mrs. F at a time when online work was not available. The possibility of online treatment now makes these situations even more complex to understand, since either party can implicate issues around online work to obscure the important dynamic meanings accompanying real-life external challenges to maintaining the work toward a good goodbye.

What Is the Therapist's Role in Middle-Phase Difficulties?

Work in the middle phase can be long, painful, and often frustrating for the analyst, as the patient clings to the closed system and tries to provoke the therapist to act in a way that pushes the patient into what Steiner has called a "psychic retreat."[9] We have pointed out that an omnipotent delusion cannot be created or maintained without the participation of the external world.[10] Our feelings and conscious and unconscious responses are part of the patient's external reality. The patient may retreat from the risks of realistic functioning for his own internal reasons, but if this reaction is too frequent or too prolonged, we should examine ourselves to see if we are contributing to the difficulty. We might be reacting to the patient's new pleasure and creativity with envy; we may be reacting to the patient's growing self-analytic competence with feelings of rejection, uselessness, or loss; the thought of impending termination may evoke worries ranging from loss of income to fears of abandonment and depression.

If we don't work through these feelings, the patient may feel, perhaps in repetition of earlier childhood experiences, unable to sustain a sense of his "true self."[11] The true self encompasses the capacities of the open system, while a "false self" is part of a defensive wish for an omnipotent capacity to care for and control a depressed or unavailable, abusive, or lost parent. If we can work through our own psychic retreat from conflicts about the patient's progression, we will be available to help the patient consolidate the possibility of an open system of self-regulation and move forward from the static timelessness of omnipotent beliefs into the pretermination phase of treatment.

A supervisee brought his difficulty with a female patient to supervision. His patient had talked about a dispute at work, and the therapist once again addressed a pattern he had discerned frequently before. At the end of the session, the patient said, "I think I talked about it differently today, and it would have helped if you had noticed and said something about it." The therapist was confused because he had not noticed the difference and felt he was being falsely accused. I suggested that he ask the patient about the difference, admitting that he may have missed something important; in any case, such an instance was important for them both to understand, particularly because the patient often felt misunderstood.

In the next supervision, the therapist described a meaningful discussion with the patient about her mother's lack of attention and support for her growth. He had realized that he had fallen into a set pattern of listening influenced by the patient's history, as well as his own uncertainty about how to handle the potential ending of her treatment. These factors had combined to render him less sensitive to her present progressive functioning.

Institutional situations often pressure therapists to start, continue, or finish patients according to external demands or criteria of training programs, internships, or residencies, rather than the intrinsic needs of the patient. Similar pressures arise from the restrictions imposed by third-party insurers, health plans, and so on.

As work progressed toward a satisfactory ending of a well-conducted child analysis, the trainee was pressured by the parents to finish soon, but his training center required him to see the case longer. In supervision it became clear that the trainee had lost sight of the child's needs and the internal needs of the parents to properly complete their work as well. Recentered on them, the trainee was able to help the parents define the remaining tasks, work with the child to consolidate the gains, and have a good goodbye.

When such external pressures arise or are built into the treatment situation, it is important that the therapist not deny them but address them with patients, supervisors, and teachers.

How Does the Therapist Support Progression between the Middle and Pretermination Phases?

There are several ways therapists can foster movement into a pretermination phase. One is a positive use of counter-reactions, where we notice our own feelings and use them to help us understand what is going on in the therapeutic relationship. Another is making use of the concept of treatment phases, helping the patient understand where the current situation stands in relation to the whole progression of the work. Third is underlining and supporting the pleasure of open-system functioning and maintaining focus on the conflict between the two systems. Fourth is staying mindful of the operation of the growth principle as it helps us define a treatment goal of restoration to the path of progressive development, whatever the age of the patient. Just as we have stressed the importance of dual goals in child and adolescent treatment, that is, including the transformation of the parent-child relationship to a lifelong resource for all, here too it is important to pay attention to fostering growth in an adult patient's significant relationships.[12]

When therapists keep the growth principle in mind, we can pay attention to the present therapeutic tasks while thinking ahead to where we are going. This is working at the leading or forward edge of the patient's capacities, both strengthening and relying on the person's increasing sturdiness.[13] Late in the middle phase of treatment, we begin to consider the patient's readiness to embark on the tasks of the pretermination phase. These will be to:

1. Maintain progressive momentum.

2. Take increasing responsibility for joint work.

3. Translate insights into action.

4. Consolidate open-system functioning and bring the possibility of choice between systems of self-regulation into the foreground.

5. Address remaining omnipotent wishes and beliefs that protect closed-system functioning.

6. Anticipate the work of termination for integration, consolidation, and mourning.

How Can Therapists Make Positive Use of Their Own Feelings?

All therapists have feelings about their patients. These feelings can be of different levels of intensity and at different levels of consciousness, and may represent a response to something that comes from the patient—a counter-reaction—or they may be connected to the therapist's own history and personality—a countertransference. Here too belong issues of the co-creation of feelings in a particular dynamic relationship.

Moves toward premature termination have to be dealt with before the treatment can go forward into a pretermination phase. Since the patient often presents the wish to end as a rational consideration based on improvement, how can the analyst differentiate a unilateral premature plan from a valid one? Often, the initial indicators appear only in the therapist's feelings.

The man who flew away in his airplane, just as he had ridden off in adolescence on his motorcycle, left us both in an idealized state of self and other. I had saved his life and performed miracles, and he was becoming a great flyer. What was avoided was the reality of disillusionment and the pain of facing the fact that neither he nor I was perfect. I learned from him and many adolescents that setting aside an omnipotent image of the self or the other is a precondition for, and a part of, a useful termination phase.

Late in his analysis, Mr. G came to the last session of the month, the day before my vacation. I waited a few minutes before noting that Mr. G had not given me the check, as was our custom. Mr. G said that he had forgotten that it was the last session of the month and then said, in a flat tone, "I guess I must be angry at you for taking a vacation." He went on to recount details of his current life events. I noted Mr. G's sliding past the question of the check, as he dutifully ran through all the transferred wishes we had uncovered, especially those of wanting to deny and destroy his envied father.

Mr. G's tone of helpless resignation and my own mixed feelings, ranging from helplessness to a wish to argue, alerted me to the possibility that Mr. G had externalized his internal conflict onto the treatment relationship. His memory lapse, the provocation of a sadomasochistic battle, and the invoking of material about his father all defended against Mr. G's experience of helplessness at being unable to control being left by his analyst/wife/mother. My vacation challenged Mr. G's omnipotent conviction of complete control. He reconstituted his omnipotent belief by turning the tables and making beloved people be the ones rejected, abandoned, and forced to feel helpless or overwhelmed. He imagined me desperately clinging to him for survival, safety, and love.

With these defenses still operating in Mr. G on return from vacation, I became aware of my own moments of sudden sleepiness, a sharp drop in awareness. I tracked those occurrences and found that they came in conjunction with material related to separation. It is useful to follow closely not only the operation of the patient's ego functions but also to monitor those ego functions therapists use for working together. I realized that my feeling was one of being dropped, suddenly feeling all alone. So at those times I began to make remarks such as, "I feel you're not here today." Mr. G responded in a definite way, "Yes. Now that you mention it, I notice that I'm talking to you, but I'm somewhere else."

This was the inception of a long, painful, halting period of work that led eventually to reexperiencing and reconstruction of his mother's reactions to any success on his part. Mr. G's mother focused her attention on him only when she worried that he had a medical condition; an able child did not need her, and she dropped him instantly. Mr. G's defensive omnipotent belief that being crippled would ensure attachment, control, safety, special powers, and sexual excitement emerged. Mr. G's withdrawal in the sessions, first picked up in my feelings of being dropped, presaged a possible premature termination, which was averted by sensitivity to my counter-reaction to his closed-system functioning.

What Are the Signs of the Transition between the Middle Phase and the Pretermination Phase of Treatment?

As experiences of joy, creativity, love, and competence become more frequent and more extended, and as pleasure and confidence in working together in treatment are more dependably present, issues of separation and loss may reappear in the form of thoughts about termination. Both patient and therapist (and the parents of child and adolescent patients) may think, separately and together, of the reality of a possible ending in the foreseeable future. Often it is in our own feelings that we first experience intimations of issues around the transition from middle to pretermination phases. The end of the middle phase is marked by a general increase in working through and collaboration, but these are not without conflict. At this point in treatment, we often find patients able and willing to work but not to get better.

The idea of a pretermination phase derives from the ongoing work throughout the treatment on the importance of thinking before acting. The therapist and patient (and significant others) have to explore together whether thoughts of ending represent predominantly progressive movement or a defensive retreat. There first must be a time without a definite plan in order to figure this out and assess readiness to begin the work of an actual termination phase. We have defined this as a "pretermination phase" and think it is an essential element of preparation for a good ending.

Mrs. T and I became increasingly skilled at spotting reversions to externalizing transferences, power plays, and sadomasochistic patterns of relating, and the intermittent operation of omnipotent, hostile beliefs in control and perfection. Mrs. T was taking on increasing responsibility for self-reflection and observation of the analytic process, and she was experiencing more pleasure in all areas. This led me to notice my own occasional thoughts that we might be moving toward pretermination. But Mrs. T made no reference to ending or even thinking about termination.

I found myself musing, occasionally sleepy, and vaguely impatient. Mrs. T began to talk about the financial burden of the treatment and suggested that there was "really nothing more going on here." She thought it was time to just stop. I was taken aback by her proposed precipitate manner of ending. My knowledge of all the important work of pretermination and termination phases helped me see that Mrs. T was seeking a premature ending.

I talked with Mrs. T about the factors that go into deciding to begin a finishing time. One important element is the patient's feelings about the relationship with the analyst—if Mrs. T had already withdrawn emotionally, it was as if there were no one left to say goodbye to. Mrs. T said angrily, "I've never been left by anyone before, so I'll make sure this is not the first time!" This allowed me to interpret Mrs. T's avoidance of love and sadness by preemptive control. She felt anxiety and the threat of helplessness in the face of loss of an experience and a person really important to her. She was afraid of having real loving feelings that were not as predictable as her closed-system unhappiness or numbness could be. Those she could control, just as she had tried to control others, including me, by provoking ill-treatment in relationships.

Mrs. T and I regained joint work and mutuality in characterizing her conflict between love and power, in effect, between open and closed systems. Looking for and articulating her real, open-system feelings about me and our work together allowed us to see a persisting omnipotent idea of emptying the analysis of dynamic activity in order to provoke me to kick her out. She could then be angry with me and avoid feeling helpless in the face of her sadness and love. She could reinstate her closed-system way to regulate her life.

In a moving session, she remarked that for days she had a melody running through her head—then she realized it was the Cole Porter song where the lyrics say "Every time we say goodbye, I die a little." She said, "I can see why we need time to work through these feelings, since now I am only concentrating on the pain." I could point out to her that we had already had many goodbyes that she had survived, also without turning into her depressed mother. Our task going forward would be to look at remaining obstacles to growing from the experience of love and sadness.

Notes

1 See J. Novick and K.K. Novick (2000) for an extended discussion of objective love and how it grows through the phases of treatment.

2 J. Novick and K.K. Novick (2016) summarize these findings and describe in more detail the model of two systems of self-regulation.

3 Schlesinger 2013. Like Schlesinger, we too see earlier phases of treatment as times when we can anticipate and try to prevent premature termination, as well as mark the process of practicing positive experiences of changes, losses, and separations on a smaller scale than the eventual termination of treatment.

4 The transference neurosis is another classical psychoanalytic concept we should reclaim. For further discussion, see K.K. Novick and J. Novick (2002) and Schlesinger (2013), who contributed an important description of the relation between transference neurosis and termination.

5 Tronick and Gianino 1986.

6 K.K. Novick and J. Novick 2010, 2011.

7 Young-Bruehl and Bethelard 1999; Anna Freud 1965.

8 See DeVito, Novick, and Novick (2000) for a discussion of the interferences that result when autonomy and separation are confounded.

9 Steiner 1993.

10 J. Novick and K.K. Novick 1996a.

11 Winnicott 1960.

12 Anna Freud 1965; K.K. Novick and J. Novick 2005.

13 Tolpin 2002.

5

Pretermination

Why Do We Need a Pretermination Phase?

Pretermination as a phase of treatment is a new idea, first described in detail as such by us in the earlier edition of this book.[1] Most authors on termination bemoan the fact that so many treatments end prematurely when an adult patient or a child's parents announce that they are stopping. This is a major cause of burnout in mental health workers, as the pain of being left repeatedly and suddenly can ultimately undermine our confidence in our clinical expertise.

From the founding of psychoanalysis more than 125 years ago, an original overarching goal of psychodynamic treatments was to change the propensity for impulsive actions (id) into words and thoughts to consider with a therapist (ego). There has been theoretical elaboration of patients' need to defend themselves from anxiety or the repetition of trauma through symptom formation and what we have described as closed-system solutions. This has deepened and enriched our conceptualizations, particularly regarding the importance of the therapeutic alliance and its role in preserving treatment from premature endings. We and our students have found these ideas and the techniques that follow from them helpful in preventing and forestalling unilateral terminations. And yet the rate of early terminations has barely decreased for many practitioners. Some schools of psychoanalytic thought privilege "the relationship" as the main or only curative factor in therapy and thus, perhaps in an excess of care not to rock the boat, do not demand a mutual commitment to the work.

What more can we do? In chapter 2, we described our practice of contracting with new patients from the beginning to follow the "working arrangements." These are all designed precisely to support the alliance and to buttress it against impulsive ending. Our provision of thirty days' notice before either party makes any change has proven to be especially helpful in this regard. Then the work of nurturing the alliance continues throughout all phases of treatment and, in the context of termination, can directly counteract impulsive action in favor of thoughtful examination of options.

In the work of the treatment, the pretermination phase brings together themes from past phases of the treatment and a reworking of aspects of the patient's history, as well as integration at deeper levels and the inclusion of hitherto undisclosed or undiscussed material. Without a pretermination period of putting insights into action, consolidating the developmental experience of the treatment, and internalizing achievements of the therapeutic alliance, there is a serious risk of confusion and misunderstanding during the termination phase. A mishandled termination can ruin the work of a good treatment.[2] With consideration of the reality of ending, we depart from the timelessness of the middle phase and actively import the reality dimensions of time and change into the situation, as these are intrinsic to the patient's original goals of changing aspects of their functioning. This allows a transformed formulation of the current problem as an internal conflict between the patient's wish to change and the forces that make them reluctant. Then each side of the conflict can be examined and worked on.

But since no date has been chosen as yet, both patient and therapist have the time and space needed to work on conflicts, anxieties, feelings, beliefs, and strengths in relation to ending. This underscores the value and necessity of a pretermination phase.

What Are the Characteristics of the Pretermination Phase in Relation to Termination?

This is a time of getting *ready* to say goodbye. The pretermination phase involves reworking themes already explored, as well as discovering new areas that have to be addressed. It emerges from a growing sense in both therapist and patient that progressive development has been restored, that there has been a change in the balance between open- and closed-system functioning. Movement and sustained momentum make ending a real possibility.

The length of the pretermination phase can vary widely because each patient is different and has a different relationship to issues of successful independent achievement, loss, and separation. This is the time when patient and therapist can assess together what remains to be done before termination work can be started.

Adult patients of all ages tend to revisit the developmental tasks of late adolescence during the pretermination phase. Setting aside omnipotent beliefs, forming and integrating realistic perceptions of self and others, forging a new relationship among the pleasure, reality, and growth principles, and making choices of partner, career, and life path are all explored anew in the pretermination phase work. It offers patients a chance to revisit and rework these late adolescent developmental choices.[3]

What Is the Therapist's Role in Pretermination?

To work effectively with the strong feelings and intense conflicts that arise, we must feel sincerely comfortable with our own pretermination tasks— to relinquish initiative without withdrawal, to allow for and acknowledge the patient's increasingly effective autonomous functioning without being overwhelmed by feelings of abandonment, loss, or defeat. We have to be able to relinquish the satisfying experience of competent use of our own egos and still feel that we are important to the patient and the work. This is a juncture at which we become newly aware of the importance of a wide range of sources of self-esteem for ourselves since dependence on the patient's neediness will cripple both therapeutic partners and bring the treatment to a standstill.[4]

Erna Furman drew on her observation of mothers and toddlers to describe a sequence of engagement that can usefully be applied to work with patients of all ages. At first, the parent does for the child, then does with the child, and then stands by to admire as the child does it herself. The fourth step describes mastery when the skill has become internalized and autonomous.[5] This simple sequence carries profound implications: we begin treatment by doing a lot of the work, showing the patient how the method will work. Then we work together through the middle phase. Eventually, in the pretermination phase, we can stand by to admire as the patient takes on increasing autonomy in the joint endeavor. By termination, patients are ready to work on their own, to be their own therapists, like Furman's fourth step.

Parents or significant others have the parallel task of enjoying and validating the patient's progression. Central to working with parents during this phase is helping them shift from the mode of doing for the child to the equally important stance of being there to validate, reflect, admire, and promote progressive moves. Formulating their tasks in these terms allows for ongoing assessment of parents' readiness to undertake the work needed to accomplish termination. Sometimes the patient is there, but parents or spouses have not caught up and need further work before termination can begin. A delay of termination with child or adolescent patients may be necessary, along with intensification of parent work. Adult patients may need focused attention on the importance of bringing the spouse into synchrony with their progress. Remaining marital conflicts sometimes surface in the treatment at this point and need to be addressed before the patient can move on.

How Do We Address the Tasks of the Pretermination Phase and What Difficulties Can Arise? What Do We Mean by "Maintaining Progressive Momentum" and "Taking Increasing Responsibility for Joint Work?"

Conflicts can emerge around each of the tasks of the pretermination phase, as we foresaw toward the end of the middle phase. Addressing the anxieties and conflicts around effective action leads to a surge of good feelings and independent therapeutic work in and out of the sessions. Increasingly independent work is another of the tasks of this phase. Tracking patients' willingness to assume increasing responsibility for the joint work, for instance, noting their own slips of the tongue, undertaking associations to dreams, noticing and wondering independently about moods or tones of voice, and so forth, reveals strengths and also the resistance to and conflicts around autonomy.

Pleasure in the functioning of one's ego, as experienced in therapeutic work itself, is an achievement of the middle phase of treatment. But this pleasure is not, and cannot be, static. Intrinsic to it is progressive momentum that carries implications of moving on in life and ending treatment. Whatever the particular content of the patient's ideas about termination, conflicts that relate to separation, independence, and autonomy in the formation of an adult self-image give rise to fluctuations in motivation for the therapeutic work.

A first sign of difficulty may be a shift in the patient to feeling that working together is an imperative imposed by the therapist, rather than a challenging but voluntary and pleasurable task. With the impetus for functioning thus shifted from ego satisfaction to superego acquiescence, the scene is set for patients to externalize their conscience. Then the therapist becomes the carrier of the motivation for progress. A clue to this change may come in the therapist's feelings, as we can find ourselves wanting to nag the patient or feeling disappointed that the patient has not accomplished some plan. The patient may feel criticized and may respond with stubbornness—both people have reverted to a closed-system tug of war.

The patient's conflicts over responsibility for maintaining progressive momentum can illuminate resistance to moving forward toward the end of treatment. Slowing down, stalling progress, or delaying ending may indicate the continuing presence of intense anxiety about separation and autonomy or omnipotent ideas of staying with the therapist forever. Once progressive momentum is reestablished through work on the components of the conflict between a wish to stay with the therapist forever and a wish to get on with life and complete the therapeutic work, the patient and therapist can look together at what remains to be done before starting a termination phase.

Following work consolidating selective identifications with the positive aspects of her psychotic mother, Mrs. K felt ready to talk about termination. I also felt she was ready and suggested we think together about what remained to be addressed. After a brief period of work on her fear of loving me and being dependent, she became depressed and claimed it was biological. She went back to the medication she had stopped using years before, with little benefit. Only after the link between her depression and the beginning discussions on termination was interpreted did the depression lift and allow her to experience sadness at the thought of leaving a long, meaningful relationship.

The open-endedness of a pretermination phase gives time and space for dealing with unexpectedly severe reactions, like Mrs. K's. It gives both patient and therapist time to work through the whole range of feelings and meanings about endings before setting a specific date.

What Is Meant by "Putting Insights into Action" and What Difficulties Can Arise?

Patients as well as therapists may take genuine pleasure in achieving insight, thinking together about aspects of the material as they arise in sessions. The proportion of the patient's input increases throughout the middle phase and is part of the readiness for pretermination. But the therapist may begin to notice that these insights are not being translated into relevant actions in the patient's life. This is one of the major tasks of the pretermination phase. It relates intrinsically to the process of change and forward movement.

A middle-aged man in treatment for years seemed to get great enjoyment and satisfaction out of the emotional and intellectual interchange, but the insights achieved did not affect his external life. Mr. J still felt deeply insecure and unfulfilled in professional and personal relations. He had suffered extreme childhood situations of abandonment and loss. As it became more evident that insights were not being put into action, his belief in his own omnipotence emerged clearly. He should not have to exert himself to get what he wanted. External pain and dysfunction was the route to keeping the analyst/mother from leaving. He said, "If my outside world improves, then what is there for us to do together? If I don't need you, you'll drop me, and I'll never see you again, and I can't sustain another loss. It is clear that being with you is more important than independent pleasure in my life."

How Do We Respond to Flare-Ups of Old Ways of Dealing with Anxiety?

We see conflict between open- and closed-system functioning in the pretermination phase in many contexts. This is a danger point for premature termination, as there may be a reversion[6] to closed-system equating of autonomy with separation, loss, and depression. The patient may attempt to avoid the pain of loss by reverting from a differentiated to an externalizing transference. The part of the patient that feels like an abandoned, lonely child may be externalized onto the therapist, who can then be left behind by the powerful patient as a parent in the transference. The first sign of such a shift can be detected in the quality of working together, as the patient may become subtly sarcastic, impatient, or patronizingly tolerant. As one patient said, "Since I can do the work without you, you're useless, and I don't need you anymore." Independent work has become perverted, made into a hostile method of control and discarding of the other. This stance can easily provoke therapists into hurt retaliation as the patient appears to be devaluing and destroying their joint work.

Sticking to the phase-appropriate task helps us stay focused on the goal of this phase of work and begin to address the patient's defensive reversion. We can first question the evident assumption that the patient's effective, independent work threatens our competence or undermines the relationship. The many forms in which this interaction appears represent anxieties from all levels of development aroused by the patient's progressive development. Thus, there are likely to be repetitions of this interaction as the patient and therapist work through profound, primitive fears of abandonment, impulses to dominate or submit, competitive and comparative concerns, shame and guilt, anxiety over differences and disagreements, and so forth.

How Are the Goals of Treatment Restated or Redefined in the Pretermination Phase?

Goals have been defined and redefined throughout treatment. But as we continue to discover and deal more effectively with underlying omnipotent beliefs, the cognitive distortions and lack of differentiation that are part of the cost of maintaining closed-system functioning become more evident. Techniques of addressing false beliefs, derived originally from psychoanalysis and now often used in cognitive-behavioral therapies, are useful here. With greater insight achieved about the deep needs served by the closed system and the beginning of open-system alternatives in place, therapist and patient can look at the concepts that have been confused and then maintained in that confused state to support the closed system. Here we can differentiate, for instance, envy and admiration, enthrallment and love, repetition and transformation, addictive high and creative joy, guilt/regret and shame/ remorse, secrecy and privacy, separation and separateness, states and signals, to name a few.

Most important in this context is the distinction between mourning and traumatic loss, abandonment, and depression. It will take the actual work of the termination phase to address the tasks of mourning. By the pretermination phase, we are looking at the patient's readiness to experience sadness and begin to mourn in the termination phase, with its new context of the reality of ending.

How Do Developmental Dimensions Enter into the Conflict between the Two Systems During Pretermination?

Older adolescents have the developmental tasks of identity formation and the integration of childhood self-images with the realities of their adult bodies and selves. In order to accomplish this transition adaptively, adolescents are faced with the necessity of setting aside childhood omnipotent images of self and others developed in the service of defense, acknowledging the loss of the associated wishes, and finding new ways to fulfill the functions omnipotent beliefs have served in their personalities. The work of the middle phase of therapy addressed interferences with ego functioning and provided insight into the underlying conflict. Yet, when those insights must be put into action, resistance invariably arises in the form of clinging to irrational closed-system solutions that protect an omnipotent self-representation. The therapeutic tasks of the pretermination phase interact significantly with the developmental tasks of late adolescence; resistances that arise to accomplishing the pretermination tasks of putting insights into action, maintaining progressive momentum, and taking increased responsibility for the therapeutic work illuminate particular aspects of conflicts that must be addressed before termination may be planned.

Mrs. M had always made her attachments to important people through a painful relationship, and this had been worked on at various points throughout her treatment. The idea of termination made it possible to bring this issue back into the center of the analytic work with renewed focus on her belief that she couldn't allow herself to flourish because I would then abandon her. Her childhood conviction that her independent, creative functioning and pleasure would lead to sudden rejection had been the organizing defense of her life, affecting her ability into adolescence to flourish in college. Planning a pretermination phase of indeterminate length in order to work as we needed to on her central anxiety was reassuring to Mrs. M; it put her in charge of what happened to her in a realistic way since she would be choosing the date only when she was ready. Then we were able to proceed to work on the conflict between the two systems and their intrinsic incompatibility within the security of a pretermination phase.

How Do We See the Outcome of Conflict between Two Systems of Self-Regulation during the Pretermination Phase?

One of the ways we have characterized the overarching clinical task of the pretermination phase is in terms of the intrinsic conflict between open and closed systems of self-regulation. We think that the pathological closed-system belief in an omnipotent self, magically able to force others to meet one's needs, derives first from the helpless child's need to deal with disappointments, deprivations, or pain in real experiences of important early relationships. It is possible, although increasingly difficult, to maintain such beliefs throughout childhood and into adolescence without external validation. Omnipotent beliefs and an omnipotent self-representation are not, however, "outgrown" or "relinquished." Instead, we articulate the therapeutic and developmental goals in terms of such beliefs being "set aside," since our experience shows that they are never entirely given up or demolished.

Young people face recurring developmental challenges throughout adolescence and recurring possibilities to choose between closed- and open-system solutions to conflict. If they continue to make closed-system choices, they may manifest a number of contradictory beliefs, for instance, that one can kill oneself and still be alive. The pretermination phase of adult treatment offers a new opportunity to do what was not fully done in adolescence, to set aside the omnipotent belief in being able to operate in both systems at once and not having to choose.

Lara, twenty-one, a highly successful student with a history of suicide attempts, struggled through the middle phase to face her fears of being lost and alone without her magic to rescue her. But over time we were able to see how expensive her magic was and assess the cost in lost pleasure, inhibited achievement, and constricted relationships. This "cost/benefit analysis" became the fulcrum in pretermination for Lara's sense of having a choice and having to choose, as well as clarifying the gains in open-system functioning.

How Does the Pretermination Phase Contribute to Evaluating Readiness for Termination?

Central to the pretermination phase is the assessment of readiness to do the work of the termination phase. Both people can assess whether the patient can work effectively away from therapy, take the initiative and work fruitfully in the presence of the therapist, share the work done, accept and work productively with the therapist's interventions, and continue to work, even amid upsurges of dysphoric feelings and defenses, and recover from them more quickly. The work reflects a more mature level of relationship and a newfound desire for mutuality and objective love rather than narcissistic exploitation, enthrallment, submission, domination, or secret gratification.

What Specific Dimensions Are We Assessing?

In discussing the further accomplishments of the pretermination phase, here are dimensions therapists and patients can be looking for:

1. Pleasure in competence and autonomous ego functioning.

2. The use of new ego skills to resolve conflicts within and to negotiate conflicts with other people.

3. Transformation of the relationship to actual or internal parents in the direction of realistic perceptions. Increasing autonomy in relationships with important others (parents, spouses, children, siblings). Integration of a realistic self-representation.

4. Quality of love between patient and therapist.

5. Neutralization: the distancing of play and work from omnipotent needs. Autonomous motivation for work and creativity, in and out of treatment.

6. Setting aside omnipotent beliefs, including the idea that one can simultaneously function in both closed- and open-system ways.

7. Internal change established as a criterion for termination, in contrast to external progress only.

8. Fulfillment of basic needs in multiple open-system relationships.

9. Registering good feelings as coming from internal and external sources.

10. Increasing delinking of separation and separateness from feared unbearable loss.

How Do Pleasure in Competence and Autonomous Ego Functioning Appear in Clinical Work?

This dimension is an important result of therapeutic work for patients of all ages. The work of treatment helps children transform their sources of self-esteem from dependence on outside or magical fantasy achievements to their own genuine competencies. The coalescence of conscience further provides for a shift from outside to inside, with praise from an internalized superego supplying additional good feelings. These developments show in children's increasing pleasure in work, both in and out of treatment, and in their enhanced capacity to enjoy playing cooperatively and applying the same rules to everyone. These achievements of the school years correlate to adults' open-system relationships to work in and out of treatment.

By the time Robert was seven, there had been consistent good reports from home and school for some time. In treatment, he had been engaged in an extended period of fruitful work. He spoke of having few problems left and wondered what would happen when they were all gone. Termination was clearly on everyone's mind, and the possibility was raised by his parents. I felt that Robert's self-esteem was sufficiently rooted in real achievements to allow for thinking about the beginning of a termination phase. Tracking fluctuations in the therapeutic relationship led to our understanding of Robert's secret belief that he alone kept both me and his mother powerful and alive by being a baby with problems. When I interpreted Robert's wishful maintenance of this idea, he confronted his mother with her part in going along with his staying a baby, by her acceding, for instance, to his tyrannical food fads. His mother accepted Robert's reproach, and used my support to tell him that she wanted him to be a big boy and that she and daddy enjoyed his big boy achievements. With this he took a further leap forward.

With renewed self-confidence, Robert told me that he had been able to put his face in the water while swimming. He alluded repeatedly to a wish to finish his treatment. I agreed that he was ready but said that I would leave it up to him to suggest when, so that we could talk about that. Robert worked in that very session to begin choosing a date but asked me to tell his mother, "because she'll be frightened out of her wits, and you know what wits are. Wits are the widths in the swimming pool, and she is so frightened, she can't even swim a width, but I can swim a whole width!" When we reached the waiting room, Robert proudly announced that we were ready to decide which day to finish.

In Robert's material and his approach to finishing his treatment, we can see the shift in his sources of self-esteem, played out in his increasing pleasure and competence in working together. The new flexibility of his ego functioning appears in his enjoyment of wordplay, even in the midst of strong feelings about his mother's worries. He showed increased self-confidence in his swimming and was brave enough to articulate his accurate perceptions of his parents' continuing anxiety over his growing up. Work with his parents was needed to help them reach Robert's level of confidence in his consolidation at the new level of development, but soon we all agreed that the treatment would end in three months.

In adults, we similarly look at their capacity for mutuality, acceptance of their realistic feelings of admiration for the analyst, and competent exercise of ego functions in evaluating impulses and wishes.

How Does the Patient Begin to Use New Ego Skills to Resolve Conflicts Within and Negotiate with Other People? How Does This Relate to the Development of the Self-Reflective Function That Is Considered a Goal of Treatment?

As patients begin to move toward independence and ownership of themselves, old fears may be revived. Patients may rush to leave treatment, either concretely or symbolically, to avoid their own issues around leaving and the pain of mourning. At this point, we need barometers of readiness to have a good goodbye. Because the therapeutic alliance tasks are internal to the treatment, therapists and patients can together assess how much they are taking responsibility for working together, how well they are able to continue to move forward despite occasional setbacks, and how much they are able to own their increasing pleasure in work and play both inside and outside the therapeutic relationship.

> Mr. M, who took a long time to pick a date, struggled with his conflict over his growing self-analytic skills. This showed up particularly whenever he returned from a weekend or a vacation. He would describe his thinking during the absence and then somehow not draw the conclusion. He kept giving me an opening to make the point, be the one who achieved the insight. Mr. M seemed to blank out the capacities we both knew he had. The major locus of work was first within me, to retain my knowledge that Mr. M truly had these capabilities and not to intervene unnecessarily. The important clue was my own feeling of exceptional clarity, memory, and competence. On his part, he alerted me to the potential problem by saying, "I continue to be amazed that you can remember stuff we talked about years ago." Work on this externalization of his own "amazing capacities" allowed us to move forward.

How Does the Pretermination Phase Allow for Increasing Autonomy in the Relationship between Child and Parents? What Happens between Adult Patients and Their Internal Representations of Their Parents? How Do We Assess Internalized Parenting Functions in Adults?

There are many ways that parents are affected when their child develops into a more separate and autonomous individual, whether under ordinary circumstances or in the context of gains from treatment. Some parents grow alongside their child, with dynamic changes in all family members. Others use their work with the child's therapist to gain insight into their own problems; seeing the child as a separate person may enable them to seek further help for their own difficulties. Some parents feel threatened by the child's development of genuine psychological autonomy, worried that the child's differences from them imply criticism of their values or personalities, or that the child's more independent conscience topples the parents from the position of all-powerful arbiters.

More malignant is the fear that the child who functions more independently will no longer meet parental emotional needs. In families that maintain psychological equilibrium on the basis of parental externalizations onto the child, treatment gains involving the rejection of externalization and the child's coalescence of an integrated identity can destabilize the family and lead to premature termination. It is important to work with the parents' side of the conflict over separateness. In adult patients, transference manifestations of this dynamic with parent figures through enactments in and out of treatment can provide tenacious resistance to forward movement.

As thirteen-year-old Tommy began to progress, he became more aware that "they put the bad on to me, and then they feel good." As he overcame his primitive fear of abandonment and began to integrate positive aspects of his self-image, his material centered on his mother's sadness, the chaos in his home, the madness of his family members, and his own intense feelings of guilt. He was not guilty about his newly attained level of functioning itself, but rather that he had deprived the family of a vehicle for externalization. The more Tommy's positive development became apparent, the more his family was thrown into chaos. It took a long period of intensive and arduous work with the parents to help them come to terms with new ways of being together with their children.

Professor N worked long and hard to come to grips with a crippling inhibition of his academic work. After some time in treatment, he was struggling to write a grant proposal when he dreamed of sending it in with blank pages. He described the terror that infused the dream and the time after he woke up. Associations brought him to memories of "going blank" when his psychotic mother raged and ranted. I asked him about the impact those times had on his schoolwork. After a long silence, he described, in a wondering tone, that his mother used to help him fill up the blank pages of his notebooks with illustrations for his reports that they clipped together from magazines. This moving memory was the first positive recollection of his mother that Professor N had ever brought into the therapy. After this point, he was able to complete his grant proposal and began to think about his mother's gifts, as well as the poignant disability of her mental illness.

How Does Transformation of the Relationship to Parents Relate to Termination Readiness?

Late adolescence is the time for a developmental shift in the relationship between parents and children, as young people become equals, responsible to and for themselves as the source of their wishes, desires, pleasures, and competencies. Parents have the corresponding developmental adjustment to make as they transform their relationship into respect and admiration for the autonomy and independence of their child. Adult patients have rarely negotiated these passages in a healthy fashion in their own adolescence.

These transformations take effort under ordinary circumstances; for families with a young person in treatment, they are often hard to accomplish because of pathological interferences. At pretermination, as autonomy and self-generated pleasure are increasingly present in the therapeutic work, family problems over separateness are thrown into relief. Often it is only during the pretermination phase that a family's wish to terminate the treatment on the basis of external criteria appears. With adolescents in treatment, the family's goal may be physical separation at the culturally determined time, without regard to assessing internal transformations of relations to self or others. Therapists who share cultural assumptions with their patients, as most do, risk colluding with such treatment plans.[7]

What Is the Relevance of the Quality of Love between Patient and Therapist?

We have written about the pervasive denial of objective love between patient and therapist because of the confusion between love and sex, love and enthrallment, love and rejection, and so forth.[8] It is obvious that the nature of feelings between the two people will affect the termination work and the quality of life after treatment.[9] During the pretermination phase, we look together at the quality and constancy of the patient's regard for the therapist. This has been implicit in the emotional tone of being together and working together, but it must be recognized explicitly in relation to the patient's willingness to love and be loved in a mutually enhancing, respectful way. Saying goodbye to someone valued in this mature way is sad but not devastating; it is painful, but the pain is offset by good memories; the experience of mourning in a good goodbye can lead to growth.

This is a moment when it is sometimes useful for the therapist to recount memories of separations and reunions with the patient, noting with confidence their joint capacity to use those constructively. In contrast, saying goodbye in the context of an abusive, exploitative relationship carries no sadness but perpetuates trauma and leaves the individual depleted, furious, and searching for revenge by any means. To avoid such disruptive, painful states, a patient can defend against mourning by blunting all positive feelings about the treatment and the therapist.

Where Does the Therapist's Love for the Patient Belong during the Pretermination Phase?

Only in the context of love and respect for the patient as a separate person can we hand over initiative and responsibility. Awareness of the distinction between the two systems of self-regulation allows us to feel objective love— love of the real skills of self and other used separately and together, love of the work accomplished, and love for the unique, capable person the patient has become. Only with security in objective love can we also experience and use our real anger at the patient's desperate attempt to fall back on omnipotent manipulation to destroy the therapeutic achievement and the competent skills of each partner.

> I felt increasingly worried about Ms. D, whose enormous gains from therapy seemed to disappear before our very eyes as she began to have trouble at work and in her relationship with her boyfriend toward what I thought was the approaching end of the pretermination phase. I was

assailed by doubts about the efficacy of our work together. Then I began to feel irritation and frustration. Examining this signal of anger in myself produced understanding and better tolerance. More importantly, I was able to identify my signal anger as a response to Ms. D's attempt to enact an organizing omnipotent belief. Ms. D said, "If I just persist for long enough, finally, you will take care of me and be my mother; I'll make you tell me what to do, and I'll never have to leave you." She was trying to involve me in her omnipotent attempt to avoid sadness and force love in the controlling way her parents had.

I told Ms. D that I didn't like her pushing me around in this way, trying to force abandonment of our true relationship and our experience together of her autonomous capacities. I pointed out that she could make her own choices, which I would respect whatever they might be, but I would not distort or collude in destroying what we had learned together of her strengths. Externalization, even of positive qualities, does violence to the other, and I would not let her attack me and our work in this way. This confrontation led to gradual improvement. She had a long way to go, but she maintained her progressive momentum at her second attempt to move from pretermination into a termination phase.

What Contributes to Neutralization, the Distancing of Play and Work from Omnipotence?

One of the hidden costs of closed-system functioning is the degree to which the person's talents, skills, and emotional and intellectual capacities are co-opted into the service of maintaining omnipotent beliefs and sadomasochistic interactions. Patients and those around them are thereby robbed of the full flowering of potential. Wit is distorted into sarcasm, fantasy is perverted into obsessional preoccupation, generosity is corrupted into self-serving calculation, and so forth.

A patient's changing capacity to play signals a profound shift in the therapeutic relationship. For children, this is a literal assessment. How a child plays provides us with a perspective on progress toward an internalized capacity for a pleasurable, respectful relationship with self and others. With adults, this is demonstrated in an increased capacity to enjoy exploring, imagining, and considering alternatives, in greater freedom, flexibility, and creativity of thought. The importance of this aspect of therapeutic progress becomes clear when we understand that true play demands a secure arena that can only be established when there is safety and pleasure from competent, realistic functioning and relationships, the kind of working well together that grows through treatment.

It is a difficult task to put the insights of the middle and pretermination phases into action, to move from exercising capacities to sustain omnipotent functioning to using those gifts and skills in the service of realistic satisfaction and growth over time. The differences and contradictions between the open and closed systems become ever clearer, and the patient realizes the choice that is becoming available.

Mr. K, a musician who had been a child prodigy, talked during the pretermination period of listening to music in a new, deeper way, relishing the structure and resolution. He had always before found the end of a piece almost unbearable, as it made him terrified of death. Whenever he had listened to a recording, he had started the piece over as soon as it finished, so that in his head, the music became an endless loop, a denial of time and death. As he worked on tolerating his anxiety and recognizing his wish to change reality, he realized why he had given up playing his instrument before starting therapy; he had been willing to sacrifice the potential joy of performing in the service of maintaining the magic omnipotence. This work led him to resume playing.

Mr. K gradually translated the insights of the clinical work into his own theory of what he called "hard and soft technique." He said that soft technique is "what you have as a child prodigy. You are not aware of technique; you just have it, like breathing. When others respond with amazement, you too are amazed, and you take it as a sign of being special. Some time during the teen years," he continued, "soft technique has to be transformed into hard technique, or you lose it. Hard technique requires more than practice, though work is an important element. It requires reflection, owning the technique, and being responsible for its breadth, depth, and limits. Hard technique brings you to the joy of mastery and the joy of never being bored but always having more to learn. Soft technique is used for applause, but hard technique is used for a respectful, loving relationship between you and the music."

Why Is It Necessary to Set Aside Omnipotent Beliefs before Starting a Termination Phase?

The therapist's sense of being dropped, rejected, or treated with contempt is often a signal that the patient has reverted to an externalizing transference. With this comes the danger of a sudden, unilateral termination. Such a moment can also provide an opportunity for deepened work on central issues. Pretermination makes space for revisiting and enriching the understanding of themes that have recurred throughout treatment.

As we talked about choosing a date, Mr. G initiated a crusade to prove that he could force me to feel and be a certain way. He became sarcastic and dismissive of anything I said and talked about how he might as well just stop treatment now and leave me behind "crying in my beer." He sensed impatience in me, expressed his fear that I would kick him out, and then said he would be devastated and destroyed. I commented that we seemed no longer to be functioning as two adults working together to help him get ready for the next phase but had shifted into a magical, destructive system where each of us had been given life and death power over the other. This helped him gain perspective on his destructive rage. He said that his anger had made him forget how much time we had spent together and how much he had come to value thinking things through with me. Mr. G felt he was acting like the helpless two-year-old who was suddenly removed from his parental home and sent to live with strangers because his mother had been hospitalized.

Through this work, Mr. G arrived at the core of his omnipotent belief that his pain and rage could make his mother be a good-enough provider for his developmental needs. "So there it is," he said, "I have to put aside the idea that my mother could love me in the way I needed and get on with all the good things I now have. Or I can destroy all that I have worked for and go on thinking that there is something I can do to force them to do my bidding. You said there is a lot of work to saying goodbye. I can feel that now, but I think I'm ready to do it."

How Do You Establish That Change Is Really Internal?

There can be intense pressure from parents and schools to finish children's treatment when they have shown outwardly visible changes. Symptom abatement and diminution of anxiety are usually rapid after the start of treatment. These, however, do not necessarily reflect the conditions inside the child.

During the pretermination phase, ten-year-old Erica talked about wishes and how she always thought of two sets of wishes, the "baby ones" and the "grown-up ones." She wanted to tell the grown-up wishes first: they were to be a ballerina, to do pottery, to play a musical instrument, and to have four monkeys and two cats. I wondered if she had the wish to be grown up, get married, and have babies, like she used to talk about. Erica replied, "That's a baby wish because I can't work to make it come true now. I used to have it when I was doing poorly at school—I would think to myself that grown-ups don't go to school and so I wish to be a grown-up. The baby wishes were to have a magic wand, to have wings, and to be a grown-up." We see in this material clear indications of Erica's increased pleasure in her own capacity to use her reality testing to distinguish between magic and real possibilities. Ego pleasure in the work of treatment ensures an adaptive response to the hard work remaining to be done during termination. Erica and I could feel confident that she was at this point ready to pick a date.

Similarly, the tasks of the therapeutic alliance allow us to measure progress along internal dimensions, as they cannot be accomplished without change in the patient's access to and use of ego functions to engage in open-system solutions.

What Do We Look for in the Patient's Life Outside Treatment?

In the course of therapy, important ego needs have been recognized and met through the therapeutic relationship. The needs to be felt with, listened to, understood, validated, and admired for progressive achievements are basic to everyone. All partners in treatment should address the question of who will fulfill these legitimate needs for the patient when the therapy ends. Can the child elicit an appropriate response from important people in their life? Can the patient find people who will be empathic, loving, and willing to share their feelings? These basic human needs can be met by parents, friends, mentors, spouses, and partners. Final resistance to ending therapy may appear as a reluctance to put the insights of treatment into action by seeking appropriate people or eliciting needed responses from available people. If the therapist remains the only person the patient can really talk to, then a major area of resistance, probably in both people, is affecting progressive movement and must be addressed.[10]

> Mr. M had idealized me at times throughout the treatment but gradually felt the pleasure available in a more equal partnership between two competent adults. At one point in the pretermination phase. he said, "I can feel myself losing the sense of who you are. Once more you're becoming this billboard-size figure. Once more I feel that only you can give me what I need." In his fear of abandonment he had reverted from attunement to externalization and lost track of the personal resources in the rest of his life. His quick retrieval of connection to his real resources and to a working relationship with me helped us move forward.

Are "Tapering" and "Weaning" Good Models for Termination?

Many patients, as well as parents of child and adolescent patients, say that they would not want to go "cold turkey," but would rather reduce the number of sessions per week or month. Often, they liken this approach to weaning, "like cutting out the nighttime feed," said one mother. Many therapists go along with this idea without questioning the underlying assumptions and beliefs. Some patients create a gradual decrease without discussion by missing sessions or becoming very busy. The latter is especially true with child and adolescent patients, who become very busy with a variety of extracurricular activities. How can the therapist question the family's choice of after-school soccer rather than therapy when the interest in sports is the result of successful therapy? Similar dilemmas may hold true with adult patients as well.

Psychotherapy is based on a conviction that thought and discussion about an issue, rather than immediate action, are the way to bring about positive short- and long-term benefits. The whole idea of a pretermination phase rests on this assumption. This concept has guided the work through all the earlier phases of treatment; over time, the patient has come to realize that thinking and then talking is a powerful, lifelong skill for coping and mastery of the inevitable difficulties and challenges of life. It is understandable that, as an end approaches, patients may feel the pull to revert to an apparently safer, closed-system solution in which action is believed to be powerful enough to control others and avoid painful reality-based feelings, such as sadness and disappointment. Therapists, too, may revert to closed-system beliefs as they collude with the patient, equating the experience of therapy to dependence or addiction, thereby avoiding mastering the powerful and intense feelings of sadness accompanying a good ending to joint work.

When I did not immediately go along with Ms. L's plan to end her treatment by changing to a monthly schedule right away, she became very angry. After several sessions of ranting and threats to quit immediately, she stepped back and wondered why she was generating so much heat. Then she noted, "It's obvious. We're talking about separating, and we know how hard it was for me to take each growing-up step. From preschool to graduate school, I panicked each time, with stomach aches and rage." We explored once more her way of leaving home after high school, how she chose a college far from home and spent the summer before leaving in a rage at her mother, staying out all night, engaged in dangerous sexual behavior and risky substance abuse. It took more pretermination work on all the meanings of the different ways of leaving before Ms. L was able to choose a date. Much of the work involved turning our minds together to understanding her seemingly reasonable plan to wean herself from treatment. In order to have an ending that did not repeat or avoid her traumas but fostered mastery and growth, Ms. L decided to stick it out and work intensively to the end.

In this situation, the weaning model would have colluded with her defensive efforts to avoid the realities of ending. There may be other treatments where, for reasons of history or circumstance, more flexibility is indicated. Our major point here is to underscore the importance of exploring the meaning of termination plans, rather than going along with any formulaic format.

What If Therapist and Patient Do Not Agree on Readiness for Termination?

Sometimes patient and therapist cannot find their way to a shared perspective on readiness to terminate. The patient may feel the analyst is holding them back, with or without cause; the therapist may feel the patient is blind to continuing problems or to the opportunities intrinsic to a planned, mutually agreed termination. It is helpful to find a solution that does not leave both people feeling angry and adversarial, one that will leave the door open. In such instances, we often recommend a "pause" in treatment. Earlier, in describing types of endings in chapter 1, we wrote about a "pause, or intermittent treatment." This can be a fallback position for the therapist to take if the patient insists on ending when the therapist thinks more treatment is indicated.

How Do You Decide to Start a Termination Phase?

Criteria for starting a termination phase are not clear-cut or definitive. In that way, they are similar to the criteria for starting pretermination, but they are perceived by this time with greater conviction and confidence. There is more hope, as the ratio between closed and open solutions to conflict has changed markedly. The determination depends in part on intuition, a clinical sense of momentum, an assessment of resilience, and therapists' work on their own counter-reactions and countertransference needs to cling to the patient. Shared focus on the tasks of each phase provides a consensual, experience-near basis for all parties to the therapy to come to a mutual decision that the time is right to start the difficult, rewarding task of saying goodbye.

How Do You Pick a Date?

The termination period is defined as the time between picking a definite date and ending on that date. We suggest that the patient pick a date, sharing our experience that termination requires sufficient time for the work, but that too much time can obscure the reality of ending. When the patient initially suggests a date, we ask for associations, as the first try may turn out to be a relative's birthday, the day before a major event, or the day before the therapist's vacation—a day that would overshadow the ending of treatment as an important time in itself.

Often, the responsibility of choosing a date causes a resurgence of conflict. Focusing on the therapeutic alliance tasks of the pretermination phase can highlight these dynamic issues. Resistance to examining the conflict in order to avoid actively choosing a date puts the work squarely back in the realm of the conflict over progression. Maintaining progressive development implies change over time, which challenges the omnipotent denial of change, growth, generational differences, and mortality. Slowing down is a shared experience of trying to turn back the clock, which presages the work to come on omnipotent wishes to deny the reality of time. Trying with fiendish ingenuity or agonizing delay to provoke the therapist to set the date illuminates issues of independent, autonomous responsibility. Taking increasing responsibility for the joint work runs counter to the omnipotent belief that a sadomasochistic relationship of dominance and submission is the only safe and effective way of functioning. Translating insights into action challenges the omnipotent belief that there is no difference between thought and action, between fantasy and reality.

Once the date is chosen, and a little time has been devoted to ensuring that the date can truly stand on its own, the termination phase can begin.

Notes

1 J. Novick 1976, 1982; J. Novick and K.K. Novick 1990; J. Novick and K.K. Novick 2006.

2 Craige 2002, 2005; Tessman 2003; Kantrowitz 2015.

3 Ferraro and Garella (2009), in noting our contribution around the connection between adolescent leave-taking and termination, also describe the reexperiencing of trauma in adolescence through the process of nachtraglichkeit, or deferred action. For a more detailed discussion of deferred action, see J. Novick (1999).

4 It is our impression that many therapies extend well beyond their useful life. Freud noted that therapy is a cure by love: we suggest that, in our two-systems model, we emphasize the importance of the growth over time of objective love between therapist and patient as crucial for change. This approach posits that the therapeutic alliance and love in the real present relationship derive from and foster open-system functioning. These factors are at least as important as the transference aspects of the relationship. Here we are aligned with Schlesinger's minatory description of the problems around a shift from clinical therapy into a gratifying self-perpetuating relationship for both patient and therapist ([2005] 2013).

5 E. Furman 1992.

6 We use the term "reversion" rather than "regression," as the closed-system response remains a potential solution forever; addictions are not obliterated.

7 DeVito, Novick and Novick 2000; K.K. Novick and J. Novick 2023.

8 J. Novick and K.K. Novick 2000.

9 In the termination literature, there is disagreement not only about the importance of having an explicit termination phase or process but also about whether there is any difference between the treatment of patients from the ordinary population and the treatments that are usually a required part of clinical training. Studies have described the high proportion of psychoanalytic students who end their own treatments with feelings of disappointment. We suggest that this may be related to insufficient attention to termination, as these students, unlike ordinary patients, will continue to have an ongoing relationship with their analysts, sometimes for the rest of their lives, as colleagues working together in professional organizations. Craige 2002, 2005; Tessman 2003; Schlesinger 2014; Kantrowitz 2015; Salberg 2010; J. Novick 1997.

10 The interpersonal school in psychoanalysis has helpfully underscored the importance of these real relational needs in therapy. Patients described in Salberg's 2010 volume express the feeling, "Why end treatment when the relationship is so gratifying to all my important needs?" The model we propose here offers an alternative.

6

Termination

How Do You Describe the Termination Phase?

The termination phase starts when the date has been set by patient and therapist, and it ends on that agreed date. The reality of these external markers differentiates this phase of treatment from earlier ones. If the timing is right, if the phase is started not when the treatment goals have been achieved but when progressive forces are ascendant, then the termination phase can be a most stimulating and fruitful period of work for both people. The reality of an ending date also intensifies and revives conflicts.

The overall aim of the termination phase is to consolidate open-system functioning, which includes the capacity to be with another and oneself; the capacity to work together with another and alone in the presence of the other in a creative, mutually enhancing way; the capacity to be autonomous without having to separate and to retain autonomy when separate; the capacity to engage with the reality of self and others;[1] the capacity to say good-bye in a mutually enhancing way, acknowledging mourning and so internalizing the positive aspects of the relationship. These all contribute to a good goodbye.

The possibility of open-system functioning has been a goal of treatment from the start. The extent of open-system functioning has been assessed together during the pretermination phase and will now be tested, strengthened, and consolidated under the stress of a real, immutable ending date.

At the same time, the therapeutic alliance is at peak efficiency, and open-system solutions are increasingly available, offering more resources to resolve conflicts and work through potentially traumatic events. The termination phase is a time when the therapeutic achievements can be seen and tested. A wide range of affects can be experienced, owned, and used as signals and guides to further action. Feelings of disappointment, disillusionment, and sadness are particularly intense during this time; detailed work on defenses against and working through these emotions allows the patient to mourn and grow from the experience. In particular, the loss of the therapeutic relationship can be mourned, and the skills acquired through mastery of the therapeutic alliance tasks internalized as a capacity for creative living.

What Are the Tasks for the Patient during the Termination Phase?

1. To consolidate a preponderance of newly acquired or reactivated competent, open-system functioning with conflict experienced over the pull to old, closed-system omnipotent solutions.

2. To work through revived conflicts in the context of saying good-bye.

3. To more fully set aside closed-system beliefs in omnipotent power to control others.

4. To mourn the loss of the unique relationship, setting, and ways of working established in the treatment.

5. To internalize the loving, supportive, and ego-enhancing aspects of the therapeutic relationship.

What Are the Therapist's Tasks during the Termination Phase?

1. To allow the patient's realistic sadness, grief, and mourning.

2. To deal with our own sense of losing an important relationship and a unique opportunity to exercise our skills.

3. To work right to the end and not give in to pressures from within and without to alter the way of working and the nature of the relationship.

Are There Tasks for Parents or Significant Others in the Patient's Life during the Termination Phase?

In the pretermination phase, we looked at who would meet the essential needs discovered, articulated, acknowledged, and fulfilled with the therapist, such as the needs to be attended to, valued, respected, admired, and loved. Once it has been established that such people exist in the patient's world, we pay attention in the termination phase to their reactions to the imminent termination of the treatment.

Parents of child and adolescent patients are directly involved with the analyst and the therapy, and they too have to mourn the loss of an important relationship, consolidate their gains, and, in so doing, support and facilitate the child's continued growth.

Adult patients have significant others who have had a similar, though less direct and obvious, relationship with the therapist and the therapy. It is important to keep in mind that they are also ending a meaningful relationship; how they respond to the ending can facilitate or hinder further growth on the part of the adult patient. The patient is the person who does the work with the significant others, but part of the joint work of the patient and therapist during this phase is to look together at what is going on. They can address how patients can assist a spouse, friend, boss, or parent, or how the patient may be neglecting others or enacting conflicts with them.

Mrs. T began to report that she and her husband had been having long, deep talks about their lives, their relationship, and their experience of parenting. This was a major shift in their functioning together, and both she and her husband saw this as a gain from treatment. At times during the termination phase, when Mrs. T struggled to stay with her painful feelings, he would comment on her withdrawal and wonder with her if it had to do with the end of a therapeutic relationship that had become very important to them both.

Is There a Standard Way of Dealing with Termination?

There is a wide range of practices and approaches to termination, even among clinicians of similar orientation. The variability is greater than at any other phase of treatment. Beyond the fact that there has been no conventional or established standard for a termination phase, we think there are particular causes for such variability.

What Are the Reasons for Such a Variety of Styles in Termination?

Termination brings out intense feelings in therapists. In our teaching, consulting, and supervising experience, we have seen surprising, uncharacteristic behavior and blind spots even in experienced analysts during this phase, which could indicate the presence of powerful countertransference conflicts and defenses.

For example, there may be a sudden shift to self-disclosure when this was not part of the regular technique earlier in the treatment. Therapists may resort to management rather than engage in mutual exploration. Sometimes the analyst withdraws preemptively, and there ensues a loss of affective intensity or vitality, with both patient and therapist feeling that there is nothing left to do or say.

> I was pleased about the beginning of the termination phase in the treatment of Mrs. F. She talked one day about how her family was making the choices about her teenager's entry to high school. I was surprised to find myself on the verge of telling her where my children had attended and how we had weighed the different factors, since such self-disclosure had not been part of the treatment before. There was some internal pressure to rationalize the impulse on the grounds that the relationship had reached a more realistic basis. Thinking about this after the session, I realized that I was going to miss hearing about Mrs. F's children, whose development I had followed for some time. I was saying good-bye not only to this patient but to her whole network of relationships, which had become part of my mental landscape.[2]

Why Does Termination Arouse Such Intense Reactions?

Freud and his successive waves of students were brilliant thinkers and superb clinicians, yet they long ignored termination as a theoretical or technical subject. Despite some works on the topic at the end of the twentieth century, termination remains "the Achilles' heel of psychoanalysis"[3]—the denial and avoidance of termination continues. We have written before about historical, political, and personal psychological reasons for clinicians' resistance to the topic.[4]

Psychoanalysts since Freud have emphasized the traumatic impact of early maternal loss, separation, neglect, and deprivation. Neuropsychoanalytic research provides the structural basis for the functional disturbances following maternal loss observed and reported by many.[5] Here we emphasize that termination can evoke the most powerful and deepest feelings for everyone, from an infant's potentially catastrophic reaction to being neglected and abandoned to the inevitable epigenetic sequence of separation anxieties described by Freud,[6] and to the many profound experiences of loss which accumulate as one ages.

Termination is not death, but the capacities developed throughout therapy and revisited and consolidated during the termination phase offer people the emotional muscle needed to deal with the inevitable, often unexpected challenges of the life cycle, like the death of parents, mentors, and models, debility from illness and age, one's own mortality, and historical currents, like disasters, climate change, war, migration, pandemics, and so forth.

Although the impact of separation anxieties has been recognized by many, there has been little talk of termination as a phase of treatment when powerful emotions reemerge for not only the patient but also the therapist. If clinicians help a timely termination to develop, they may have to not only respond to and contain the patient's range of separation anxieties and omnipotent defenses against them but also guard against self-protection with parallel defenses. Picking an actual date for ending introduces a real-life stressor into the clinical situation. The patient and therapist can react in both closed- and open-system ways. The overall task during the termination phase is to differentiate these two modes of response, strengthen the open-system adaptive mode, and allow for genuine conflict and choice between the two systems.

> Mrs. Y said that, although she knew me from how I was with her and the work we did together, mostly I was a shadow puppet, a dim reflection on a screen thrown by a flickering candle in her head. She would miss me and the setting, but I, on the other hand, saw her clearly and knew her more intimately than anyone else did. I watched her grow and change, and I participated in that growth and change. "Probably you will miss me more than I will miss you." After a moment's reflection, I realized that she was right, and I agreed with her.

What Is the Role of Pleasure in the Termination Phase?

We have emphasized pleasure throughout this book because pleasure is a motivator. It has also been shown to have beneficial physiological effects. Most importantly, reality-based pleasure is essential to counter the addictive power of sadomasochistic, closed-system functioning. The genuine power of closed-system solutions—the addictive, sometimes ecstatic, rush—must be acknowledged by both patient and therapist, along with the recognition that dependable, reality-based pleasures may not produce the same result. The work of the treatment has enhanced open-system functioning with its own satisfactions, gratifications, and pleasures.[7]

What Is the Role of Anger, Hostility, and Revenge in the Termination Phase?

In general, anger has an important open-system role as a signal of something a person doesn't like. The signal triggers an assessment of the situation to discern the cause of the trouble and do something about it, or to recognize that there is nothing one can do. The experience of this process is satisfying in itself, as the person feels the effective functioning of the mind working harmoniously. Anger as a state, on the other hand, is a closed-system manifestation. Overt or covert hostility, unfettered rage, and the effort at revenge are all part of the powerful network of solutions the individual may have devised during childhood or adolescence to deal with overwhelming, potentially traumatic experiences.

Retaining the idea of revenge can be a secret insurance against helplessness that patients may cling to even during the termination phase. Beyond that function, hostile and vengeful fantasies and preoccupations are exciting. There is gratification associated with the discharge of aggression. Research has demonstrated that revenge triggers the same brain centers that desire, drugs, and desserts do.[8] Most people have experienced, directly or vicariously, the internal surge of power associated with thinking of the most cutting riposte, the just deserts, and the humiliation of a rival.

Mr. Q came for treatment because he was unable to focus on his work; he described the unremittingly cruel and sadistic teasing he suffered at the hands of his siblings throughout his childhood. This material came up repeatedly through his treatment, particularly as he worked through his disappointment with his mother, who was too depressed to intervene.

These memories habitually triggered intense rage and thoughts of revenge. His exceptional intelligence and imagination had been co-opted to serve these preoccupations, even while he dealt with his omnipotent equation of thought and action by the extreme inhibition in functioning. For a long time, however, Mr. Q was not interested in getting rid of his rageful preoccupation but only in ridding himself of the inhibitions. The work of the treatment revealed the accompanying closed-system belief that he could somehow go back in time and visit revenge on his brothers and undo what had happened and its impact.

By the end of treatment, Mr. Q was very successful in his creative and demanding work, had married and had children, and felt much more comfortable with his strengths. He commented that he seldom had his old revenge daydreams. He accepted that he had better ways to protect himself; besides, his brothers were now very different, and they got along very well. "But," he said, "I do miss the charge, the jolt of adrenaline when I would think of ways to destroy them. It sounds crazy, but I'm reluctant to give that up, despite knowing what it costs in terms of the rest of my life." He went on to talk about the conflict between thought and action. "I like to think that I could really do it, and that's hard to let go of. But there actually is a difference between a daydream and an action plan. I shouldn't be so scared of the daydream that I have to shut down my mind, but I'd better watch when I get swept up into the excitement of a plan."

Does Closed-System Functioning Appear at All in the Termination Phase?

Closed-system functioning always remains a potential for both patient and therapist. Under stress, old pathological anxieties, beliefs, and reactions characteristic of the closed system can be expected. These should not be a source of panic or disappointment in either person. Earlier interpretive work has decreased the intensity of closed-system reactions and allowed for the growth of an alternative open-system response. The combination of these two factors affects the speed of recovery.

By the termination phase, open-system functioning, evidenced in the accomplishment of therapeutic alliance tasks, is at peak efficiency, but the reality of ending also intensifies the potential for omnipotent, closed-system responses. What we look for and comment on is not only the return to omnipotent reactions to control or deny the reality of ending but also access to the emotional muscle of bouncing back.[9]

In her struggles over her sadness, Mrs. T would slide into self-pity, alternating between presenting herself as a helpless person, with the idea that she could make me keep her forever if she were a mess, and angry indignation that I would not comply with her wishes. Several sessions of intense anger and anxiety followed these outbursts. She telephoned me, saying that she thought she should be put on medication. I noted that her presentation of herself as incompetent had not pushed me to change the termination date, so she seemed to have upped the ante with her insistence that her feelings were so powerful that no one could control them. It seemed like a temper tantrum. I remarked on how she was using her feelings to bully and control, as she had with her parents.

I noted again how such ideas might have seemed the only available avenue at the time she was little but wondered now what had made her feel equally resourceless in the present. Mrs. T laughed and said, "It's the same old stuff. There are no guarantees, and I do wish I could have a warranty." I wondered aloud what Mrs. T really could depend on after she finished her treatment. This material opened a path to discussion of Mrs. T's ideas about what things would be like after termination. Throughout the treatment, Mrs. T struggled with the wish to hold on to past patterns of sadomasochistic relationships that represented infantile solutions with the hope of magical gratification versus the progressive forces that represented realistic relations with others and the world.

Focus on the therapeutic alliance tasks at each phase of treatment allowed for the emergence and consolidation of an alternate system of self-regulation, rooted in pleasure from competent functioning rather than control of others. Setting aside her infantile wishes from all levels of development, including magical images of perfection in herself and others, seemed a frightening and painful loss. But the work of the earlier phases of treatment allowed for the establishment of alternative sources of security and self-esteem in realistic achievements and representations. Much of the work of the termination phase involved drawing the distinction between the illusory loss of unreal fantasy gains and the real loss of the setting, of me, and of our special therapeutic relationship. At termination, her fears became particularly intense in the face of the reality of ending.

Are There Particular Resistances in the Termination Phase?

Beyond the recurrence of closed-system solutions characteristic of the particular patient, the reality of ending confronts the general denial of change, time, and reality constraints that is characteristic of closed-system functioning. So a patient may make a vigorous attempt to get the therapist to change the date.

> Mr. G picked a date, and the termination phase began. By the next week, he mounted a major effort to get me to go back on our agreement, do away with the ending date, or at least defer it for a year. It was a powerful effort, including a weekend of binge drinking and drugs, sexual bullying of his wife, and threats to fire his entire staff. He insisted that these events proved I was wrong, that he was not ready to finish and maybe never would be.
>
> I wondered briefly to myself if I had been mistaken about his readiness to finish and then wondered aloud about the function of the furor. Did the extreme intensity indicate that he was back to fighting off the painful task of setting aside his belief that he could use his troubles to force me to do his bidding? Mr. G sighed and said he had always hated change. As a child, he turned every routine into an unalterable ritual, and now his treatment had become that protective ritual he couldn't do without. With therapy he would never grow old, get sick, or die. If he could force me to see him forever, he could imagine that he was still young and slim with a full head of hair. On his own, Mr. G realized that our mutually agreed ending date was a reality confrontation with his closed-system omnipotent belief that he could simultaneously be a loving, creative person and a sadistic bully. He was able to experience the end date as a helpful anchor point and consolidate the understanding that he couldn't have it both ways.

Should the Therapist Ever Change the Date for Ending?

We have talked about how important the reality of ending is to the experience of the termination phase. Pretermination is the right time to assess true readiness to begin a goodbye time. With Mr. G, the steadfast conviction that he was equipped to handle termination was critical to weathering the storms he produced. If Mr. G had been unable to make use of interpretation, recalibrate himself, and recover momentum as the work proceeded, a return to pretermination work for a period might have been indicated.

Life events can also sometimes interrupt the unfolding of the termination work, as in the case of Mr. R, who had set a date three months ahead when he received an unexpected diagnosis of a serious illness at a routine physical examination. His condition was potentially dangerous and required major surgery. The surgery carried its own risks, and there was also the possibility of serious postoperative effects. Under these circumstances, Mr. R and I agreed that we needed more time to explore his situation and see him through his operation and its aftermath. The surgery was successful. Mr. R made a good recovery and set a new termination date.

Are Idealizations Normal and Necessary for Dealing with Painful Situations like Termination?

Some psychoanalytic models encourage the idealization of the analyst, with the idea that this recapitulates a normal developmental phase of omnipotence and idealization of the mother and the self.[10] We have a different view. We distinguish admiration, which operates in the open system, from idealization, which is a closed-system attempt to deny the real imperfections and failings of important people (parents, analysts). Omnipotent ideas are not aimed at enhancing the real qualities of the self but rather at denying and transforming pain in the parent-child relationship, filling the gap between the inadequate and the good-enough caring person. Realistic disillusionment and de-idealization are the results of addressing closed-system, defensive idealizations.[11]

> Mr. M had a very long treatment and eventually set a termination date that allowed for a termination period of fourteen weeks. He began one of those weeks shaking with anger as he expressed his need to control and boss. "The moral is I *can* provide for myself, but the wish is you'll do it for me. I'll break down at the bottom of the street. You'll see me, and you'll come and give me the best pep talk I've ever heard. The rescue will make all the angry feelings go away. You're not a depressed, incompetent mother. Look at what you can do and you're doing it for me."
>
> Then he went back to talking about the flaws he perceived in me. "Seeing your imperfections derails me. I'm deeply ashamed, like I used to react to

my parents. I was afraid to invite my friends home. I am responsible for how you are. We're back into my feelings of shame and responsibility. Why can't I accept your imperfection? So you're not LeBron James or Tom Brady—so what?" Mr. M was able to work out for himself what was going on, but, as we saw with Mr. G above, despite all the work throughout treatment, the closed-system reactions are always there as a potential, especially at times of stress like separation.

What about Disappointment?

Disappointment also belongs in the open system. It is one of the feelings that comes from an awareness and acceptance of the realistic limitations of self, others, and life. It is extremely important to gain access to idealized expectations, as we saw with Mr. M above, and then to realistic disappointment in the therapist, the treatment, and the self. In the evaluation phase chapter, we spoke of the patient's initial fantasies and expectations of treatment. Some of these do not emerge until the termination phase or even later.

Mrs. T oscillated between comfort in staying with the reality of the imminent end and fantasies about ways she could get me to change the date, change our relationship, or change myself. A week before the termination date, she seemed somewhat quieter than usual. "I'd like to write a different ending to this story," she remarked. I recalled how much we had learned together from the characters in her stories and wondered how Mrs. T would understand a character who tried so hard to redesign the world. Mrs. T snapped back, "I don't need a character to know I can't stand disappointment!" Then she said, "I really surprised myself with that. I guess it was waiting there to come out, but I have been fighting it off. Maybe that's why I've been feeling so subdued." She went on to examine the idea of being disappointed and faced her feeling that I had not been the perfect mother she had always wished for, nor was she ever going to be the perfect person she had tried to be for so long. "Maybe now, though, I won't have to run off to have secret affairs to let myself remember that no one is perfect and that's good enough!"

Disappointment of realistic wishes and goals, however, is crucial to acknowledge. Psychodynamic treatment takes time, and there is an open-ended quality to it, particularly in the middle phase. But in the meantime, real time is passing, and there are certain real-life passages, like childbearing, parenting, career choices, and so forth, that occupy a particular window of time. Ideally, these issues will be talked about throughout treatment, but during the termination phase, patients often revisit them with the task of mourning the choices no longer available. When such realities have been kept outside the treatment, the patient and therapist have probably colluded to avoid facing potential disappointment and hard choices. If pathology or circumstance have interfered with the fulfillment of realistic wishes in those windows, both people have to acknowledge and deal with this disappointment together.

Is There a Sequence to the Tasks of the Termination Phase?

The first task is to set aside omnipotent self- and object-representations. Then the patient can engage in the effort and pain of sadness and mourning for the real loss intrinsic to changes and goodbyes.[12] Often the transition into mourning is preceded by a defense against sadness and a flight into the future by one or both people.

> Dr. W had chosen a date about three months ahead, and the first part of the termination phase was marked by intensive reworking of old conflicts over loss. A major source of pain, anger, and conflict was his experiencing the end as final proof that he was unloved and unlovable. Working through intense feelings about his mother and his former therapist allowed him to regain and consolidate a feeling of objective love for himself and for me. He began to talk of his plans, both professional and personal. At first this seemed an appropriate and progressive step. Gradually, however, the sessions became filled with ruminations about what he should do in regard to this or that hypothetical postanalytic occurrence.
>
> During Dr. W's sessions, I found myself drifting into the future, joining him in analyzing his putative conflicts. I then noticed a loss of loving feeling

for him in the present. One evening I was rereading a termination article by Judith Viorst about analysts' fantasies during the termination phase.[13] I had used her material in a number of my own papers, and I thought I was going over it for a course I was preparing. I made no connection with my patient until I found myself thinking repeatedly about the reported fantasy of an analyst thinking that his patient would meet and marry his grown-up child. Then I wondered if that was my wish for a changed postanalytic relationship. My patient and I would stay together as father and son. I realized that I was avoiding my own sadness and allowing him to avoid his; I had relinquished my objective love for him as an autonomous, accomplished person who no longer needed me. I had a fantasy that might have seemed benign and loving but was actually an omnipotent desire to continue in a position of authority.

In the next session, I said that I felt we were both working hard to avoid our feelings about ending. Dr. W sighed and said that he realized he was trying to leave me in the way he had always left everyone—without any feelings of love or sadness or loss. He went on to say that his treatment provided a chance to leave while loving and feeling loved. It would be sad, but sad is better than dead, and there is no sadness without love.

Themes of disappointment in the lack of fulfillment of initial fantasies, wishes, and expectations thread through the termination of all patients in long- or short-term therapy. Recapitulation and reworking of old issues and the history of the treatment from the vantage point of new open-system capacities are part of the weave. A mutually agreed, well-timed ending phase allows these themes to emerge and be shared.

Do We Talk about Life after Treatment?

This is a major part of termination work. It usually comes up naturally in the course of engaging with the patient's reactions during the termination phase. It is not surprising that there is a range of issues that arise, varying with each person's particular history and course of treatment. This topic usually invokes familiar themes, such as changing the nature of the relationship, the equation of separation with abandonment or death, the wish that all conflicts would be obliterated, and so forth. We routinely note if the patient fails to mention or ask about post-treatment contact.

Here are some examples of post-termination issues that arise during the termination phase:

Mr. S wanted to know if he could contact me afterward. "Should we fix a specific time, like early Sunday morning?" Then he began to laugh, as he remembered past material, in which "early Sunday morning" referred to his hostile wish to interfere with and control parental sexual activities. After this understanding of his ongoing wish to control me, I explored with him the importance of integrating his therapeutic gains with his ongoing life and the usefulness of keeping me available as a therapeutic resource to be remembered or recontacted if needed, in contrast to his former omnipotent plan to turn me into his best friend.

Often, the intense reaction to setting the ending date stems from a fear that ending is like death and there will be no possibility of contact after the analysis is through. The fear of abandonment and total loss can be disguised by the omnipotent conviction that, following therapy, the patient and therapist will be best friends, lovers, and so forth. This is especially true for those whose past experience has validated that belief. Patients with a history of abuse are particularly vulnerable around termination, and attention to responsibility, fault, blame, and motivation is needed.

Ms. E, who had been abandoned in early childhood by her father, was reunited with him in adolescence only to be sexually abused by him. As we approached the end of a long, fruitful treatment, she began talking about her research on abuse. She knew that her scientific interest was one way of dealing with her experience with her father. Then she described extending the research to boundary violations between therapists and patients. She noted how frequently this occurred and said that some professional associations accept the legitimacy of sexual relationships a year or two after the end of treatment. Ms. E quickly realized that she must be talking about us, and this enabled us to revisit her adolescent effort to deal with abandonment and loss by submitting to an abusive sexual interaction. Ms. E could encompass the reality that she had felt powerful and triumphant through her sexuality to attract and keep her father in a way she was powerless to do as a child, even while facing the reality of her father's culpability. This work allowed us to explore her reluctance to set aside the omnipotent conviction that she could control all interactions and to live with the painful, but not devastating, sadness of saying a good-bye that was neither an abandonment nor a preamble to a changed relationship.

When we work with the patient's mourning during termination, we always add that the process will continue beyond the ending and predict that it may become more intense at certain times, for instance, the usual starting time after summer vacation. We then ask about the image of the therapist at times of separation. Can the patient maintain an image of a supportive, respectful, loving person with whom they can continue an internal dialogue for restoring progressive momentum at difficult moments? We look at this issue at stressful moments during the termination phase and then add that this is what the patient will be aiming to establish after termination. We point out that an inability to maintain the positive internalized image would be a reason to recontact the therapist.

In the course of working on disappointment and disillusionment during termination, we talk about the need to differentiate omnipotent wishes that can never be fulfilled from realistic perceptions of limitations in the therapist and the method. As part of his creative self-analytic work, the patient will not only maintain progressive momentum but will probably go beyond what has already been done together. This may be a source of disappointment in the therapist, but it is important for the patient and analyst to canvass together the therapist's hope and confidence that this continued growth will occur.

> In response to a dream and my comment about continuing work after treatment, Ms. O said that her anger and disappointment were triggered when I said there would be work during and after termination. "I think I have had the fantasy that when treatment ends, there would be no conflicts left. It is a dream that when therapy ends there would be no more work. I had the hope that I could finally run back to the strong woman who would gratify my passive yearnings."

Mr. M noted near the end of his treatment, "I feel good about what I've accomplished, and I think you feel good too. But I won't stop there; I still have a lot of work to do. I know my wish to hang on to my delusions and fantasies, but I also know the good feeling of knowing what I've really accomplished and that the choices are mine. The idea that somehow the great insight will occur has passed. It's a silly idea, and if a great insight should occur, it would mean I was not ready to leave."

What Is the Role of Mourning and Sadness?

All authors agree that mourning is a major aspect of termination, but it has not been made explicit in the literature what or who is being mourned, nor how this relates to sadness, depression, or the ability to choose. Psychodynamic clinicians tend to speak about mourning the loss of a person, a phase of life, or a fantasy. In a single-track psychoanalytic theory of development, much is made of how "normal" omnipotence has to be mourned and then relinquished. With our dual-track, two-systems model, we locate omnipotent beliefs in closed-system functioning and posit that a belief is never mourned or gone but only set aside.[14] The omnipotent belief remains a potential response, but therapeutic work has helped the patient find competent alternatives and so transform a pathological belief into a wish or fantasy, a delusion into an illusion. Setting aside organizing convictions may be painful, but the pain may be likened to the withdrawal from an addictive substance. In closed-system functioning, separation is experienced as a loss of control of others and their provision of one's needs. The reaction can take the form of rage, followed by depression, which is anger turned against the self. Thus, a depressed response in defense against rage and helplessness may be an expected reaction when the patient reverts to attempts at omnipotent control.[15]

This is very different from mourning, which leads in the ordinary course to internalization and identification with aspects of the lost person and attenuates over time. The crucial issue is sadness, which is present only when there is love and when there is a genuine loss. Thus, sadness exists in the realm of the open system, with its connection to real experience. We can only mourn the loss of someone we love and, through the mourning, be able to keep aspects of the person and qualities of the relationship. What is truly mourned by both patient and analyst at a good goodbye is the unique working and loving relationship that enhanced each person and will now persist only internally as they separate. What each can internalize and identify with is a greater understanding of the realistic interdependence and independence found in a mutually respectful relationship of autonomous individuals.

What about the Therapist's Mourning?

We think analysts have tended to deny the loss we experience at the end of each treatment. Implied in the literature and in surveys of analysts' reactions to termination is the idea that an experienced therapist has worked through most of the intense feelings related to ending, except in regard to whether enough was accomplished.[16] The assumption that therapists have a neutral, professional reaction to termination is disproven by honest self-examination, open exchange with trusted colleagues, a cursory acquaintance with the widespread phenomenon of radical departures from their own standard clinical technique during termination, and a reading of Judith Viorst's classic study on analysts' fantasies at termination. In Viorst's study, the analysts reported strong, wishful, or painful reactions to case terminations.[17]

We think the notion that a good personal training analysis and years of supervised training and postgraduate experience should inoculate therapists against the pain of separation and loss represents an omnipotent defense against a dread or false belief that any such pain will lead to endless depression. With each patient, we have been privileged to know a full world of people, complex networks of relationships past and present, the characteristics of another line of work, the development of children, life passages in families, and so forth. When patients leave, in a sense, a whole world leaves with them.[18] That is worth mourning. This experience demonstrates the difference between a good goodbye and a bad ending.

Mr. C and I worked throughout his treatment on his pull to comply with his mother's anxious wishes to control his therapy and his functioning, even when he became an adult, married with a good job. Despite all the good results of our therapeutic work, he was unable at the end to withstand his mother's advice that he seek a different form of treatment and leave his work with me prematurely. I was surprised and angered by his abandonment of treatment and felt unable to mourn. Anger gets in the way of loving feelings and ordinary sadness.

In contrast, there was sadness when Mrs. E finished her long treatment. I missed her and hearing about her family, her struggles and victories, and her work and colleagues. I felt proud of the work we had done together. Over time, when something reminded me of her, I felt nostalgic pleasure at thoughts of her. This had been a good goodbye.

Another contributor to denial of clinicians' emotional experience at termination with their patients is the fact that most students enter personal treatment during training but rarely go through the same kind of termination they plan with their clients.[19] Psychotherapy, counseling and psychoanalytic students are usually treated by senior members of their local training centers, most of whom are active on the faculty and committees, attend scientific meetings, and contribute to professional life. Upon graduation, younger members become colleagues with their former analysts/therapists – a very different kind of goodbye, perhaps not really a goodbye at all. In this book and our other writings on termination, we are therefore suggesting ideas and techniques that do not match our own personal experience of treatment, nor that of our colleagues and students. We are asking each other thereby to make a leap of empathy and imagination in the service of more comprehensive, effective, and humane therapies for our patients. Learning to say goodbye in a mutually enhancing way is a lesson for one's whole life.

Is It Possible to Go Through Termination without Mourning?

The intensity, duration, and pain of mourning vary with the particular patient, the work that took place in pretermination, and the analyst's capacity to contain and support the patient's real sadness, grief, and mourning. Genuine mourning is part of an open system of self-regulation, and the sadness is balanced by hopeful anticipation, confidence, and an awareness that, through mourning, the positive aspects of the joint work can be internalized for independent continued post-treatment growth and creativity. The self-analytic functions explicitly assessed in the pretermination phase are now consolidated and available for use, if and when necessary. Included in the self-analytic capability is the capacity to assess when further help from the therapist or someone else might be useful.

The restoration of the capacity to choose and the tools forged in the accomplishment of these open-system therapeutic alliance tasks have equipped patients for the lifelong struggle against the potential to resolve conflicts with sadomasochistic, omnipotent beliefs. This is the crowning achievement of the treatment and the main outcome of the work of the termination phase.

What Happens on the Last Day?

Discontinuity in technique often appears in the last session. Therapists may have the patient sit up and have a celebratory drink—generally changing the atmosphere and stance. Our approach is to keep working as the therapist until the very end. To do otherwise would deprive patients of the relationship they have relied on and the opportunity to say goodbye on their own terms. There is much work a patient can accomplish, even during the last session, often work that will be critical to later functioning. There can be no avoidance of the reality of the end. The intensity of the last day is an opportunity to consolidate open-system feelings and functioning.

Earlier in the termination phase, we routinely ask patients what thoughts they have about the last day. As we neared the ending, I asked Mr. G about the upcoming last day. He said he was planning to bring me a gift; he wanted it to be a pleasant surprise. I acknowledged the positive feelings behind his impulse but noted that, since our work together had been about thinking and talking rather than acting, to end with an action, a surprise, was an idea worth exploring a bit more. Mr. G protested, became irritated, and accused me of being a rigid, orthodox Freudian. He then began to associate to the idea of bringing a gift on the last day. Yes, it was an expression of his love and gratitude; he had been planning to give me a book he knew I would enjoy. But it would have been a surprise, a shock, like his teenage suicide attempt that caught everyone unaware. He imagined me reading the book after the end, thinking of him and missing him. This related to his deep, painful worry that I did not like him and was happy to get rid of him. I would forget him when he was gone, and the book would force me to remember.

Ms. C began her last session by noting that she used to have many questions about me, but they no longer seemed burning. As she mused about this, she realized that her questions had been more about her—did I think she was intelligent? Did I like her? She felt she no longer needed to ask these questions either, since she felt so much more sure of herself.

She pulled out a copy of a novel that had figured largely in the treatment. The book was about the impact of wartime experiences on a young boy later in his life. She said, "I thought a lot about this and decided that I wanted to give it to you. You are the person who knows how important it is to me." I thanked her.

She had noticed on the book jacket that the author of the novel she gave me had become an important writer in his fifties. With tears in her eyes and a beaming smile, clearly talking about herself, Ms. C ended her treatment by remarking, "Some people just take longer to do it than others."

Mr. M started his last day by saying, "I feel all choked up. I've tried in the last few weeks to tell you how appreciative I am; I didn't want my feelings to pile up." He spoke of his gratitude to his wife and his parents for their support. "I'm sad and I'm excited. It's a beginning as well as an end. Sad seems to be the bigger feeling at the moment." He then brought a dream in which one of the leaders in his field makes a positive comment on Mr. M's work. "My work felt good to me and was judged good by others. That's the way I feel here. I feel good about what I've accomplished, and I think you feel good too."

He went on to recall our first meeting and the many life events he had shared with me. He wondered again about keeping in touch. "One of the things I've been thinking about is the way I used to come down on myself for not doing analysis by myself as well as I did it with you. But analysis is work; it's not easy. It was a great relief to realize I wasn't a failure for needing your skills, and now these are skills I can take with me. I feel the next few days and weeks I'll understand better what leaving means. I'm left with good memories."

Notes

1 We recognize that Winnicott's (1949) and Loewald's (1957) terminology—"objective," "objectivity," and "reality"—can be criticized as "unreflectively positivistic, naively realist, even tacitly pre-Kantian" (Barratt 1984, p. 1 I). The role of reality in much of psychoanalytic theory is a continuing problem (Rapaport and Gill 1959; Friedman 1999). It is beyond the scope of this volume to discuss the philosophical dimension, but we may at least note here the complexities in elucidating levels and kinds of reality in the psychoanalytic situation (see Modell 1989) and the history of the various ways the idea of psychic reality has been understood (see Barratt 1984). We feel comfortable with what Hanly (1999) terms "critical realism," the epistemology of common sense, science, and psychoanalysis. Hanly makes a definitive citation of Freud (1933) in this regard. Neither a single-track theory (J. Novick and K. Novick 1999), which may ignore the mutual influences of endowment and environmental factors, nor a purely intrapsychic model of motivation and cause takes adequate account of the interaction of reality and the internal life of the body and mind (M. Klein 1957). We have pointed out (J. Novick & K. Novick 1970) that Freud (1915) explicitly delineated an "original reality ego" that precedes the "purified pleasure ego" (p. 136). Levin (1994) has made a cogent critique of developmental theories that exclude the role of reality and ignore its primacy in Freud's theory. We have continued to be concerned that the rediscovery of the analyst's "irreducible subjectivity" (Renik 1993) leaves the patient prey to unsubstantiated, intrusive interpretations based on the therapist's countertransference, with the accompanying danger of denial of reality. In the twenty-first century proliferation of Kleinian-derived theoretical models, psychodynamic technique seems increasingly skewed to an almost exclusive focus on transference-countertransference phenomena, at the expense of the multidimensional, metapsychological stance that epitomizes psychoanalysis in our view.

2 Schlesinger [2005] 2013 underscored this kind of danger point for interminable treatment when the relationship takes precedence over the therapeutic work.

3 Bergmann 1997, p. 163.

4 Novick 1997.

5 Zhang et al. 2002; Shore 2002.

6 Freud 1926.

7 When we consider the difference between setting something aside and repression or dissolution, we call upon recent work by Morris Eagle that reclaims the importance of Freud's topographical model of the mind (2021). In our 2002 paper "Reclaiming the Land," we noted that much is lost if the later structural model of id-ego-superego simply replaces the topographical model of unconscious-preconscious-conscious. We suggest that addictions are not repressed but are set aside in the preconscious and can be recalled and repeated if not countered by strong alternatives developed in treatment.

8 Fehr et al. 2005.

9 Novick, K.K. and Novick, J. 2010, 2011.

10 The work of Kohut and the schools of self-psychology and relational psychoanalysis are relevant here.

11 It is always important to remember that even well-attuned parents achieve that state approximately 30 percent of the time, and work with their infants to repair the mismatches inevitable in the rest of their shared experience. See Tronick and Gianino 1986.

12 Here again, we are supported by the work of Schlesinger ([2005] 2013), who stresses that there is no change or progression without a corresponding sense of loss and its attendant emotions.

13 Viorst 1982.

14 For a more detailed discussion and comparison of conceptualizations of omnipotence, please see Novick, J. and Novick, K.K. 1996.

15 We are struck by Jonathan Lear's 2022 suggestion that Freud should have entitled his study of these matters "Mourning OR Melancholia," rather than linking them with "and." This captures Freud's contention that melancholia (now called depression) is due to a failure to mourn.

16 Firestein 1982.

17 Viorst 1982.

18 Some developmental theorists have begun to describe therapeutic work in terms of non-linear dynamic systems theory. They too describe an experience of loss at the end of treatment, when the "patient-constructed self" of the therapist departs with the patient. See, for instance, Coburn 2000, p. 764.

19 There continues to be controversy within psychoanalysis on this point, with some insisting that there is no difference between "training analysis" and "civilian analysis," while others point to numerous distinctions. For further discussion, see Kantrowitz 2015; Novick, J. 1997; Novick J. and Novick, K.K. 2006.

7

Post-Termination

What Is the Post-Termination Phase?

Post-termination is not, strictly speaking, a phase of treatment, but much of the work of therapy is shaped by its goals and measured by the quality of life afterward. Therapy is not an end in itself. It is a means to restore or establish the capacity to choose between open- and closed-system solutions to life's challenges. It includes Anna Freud's therapeutic goal of restoration to the path of progressive development. Implicitly, the entire treatment has been a preparation for post-termination living.

What Are the Patient's Tasks in This Phase?

The patient's task on the completion of treatment is to use the internalized open-system alliance capacities and skills for living and creativity.

What Are the Therapist's Tasks after the Treatment?

The clinician's post-termination task is to maintain the stance as the patient's therapist, despite internal or external pressures to alter the relationship.

Continuing positive growth after treatment is only possible when there is continuity between the time of therapy and afterward. Many patients have had the fantasy image of therapy as something terribly painful to be endured in return for a subsequent prize, such as perfect happiness, conflict cessation, or an ongoing, altered relationship with the analyst as a friend, spouse, or lover. Therapists, too, have fantasies of post-treatment contacts or changes. These have to be worked through during the pretermination and termination phases if the termination is to be truly constructive.

Is There Change after the End of Therapy?

The date of ending treatment is real and signals the end of regular contact between patient and therapist. But if the treatment has been effective, we expect the process of change to continue. Within a two-systems model, change continues throughout life, with each phase influencing each other phase in non-linear fashion, forward and backward over time. Open-system solutions continue to evolve and new access is part of growth. Equally, conflicts and closed-system solutions are never completely gone; they remain as a potential choice at times of stress.

Mr. L, a child of Holocaust survivors, whose father died when he was an infant, left analysis pleased about the changes in his life but immensely sad that he was still himself. He wrote to me two and a half years later: "The analytic process continued very actively for many months after the analysis, and it is only recently that I feel I have reached the natural conclusion of it as a distinct part of my life and as a distinct method of investigation of problems."

Mr. L described thinking about his recurring image of a child on a flinty road trying to catch up with a man who may or may not be his father. He described how, in the course of his self-analysis, he realized the whole point of the image was never to catch up with the father, to seek out failure, because failure meant pursuit but never catching up, and never catching up meant his father is not dead; he's there, ahead somewhere. He wrote that it took years after the treatment to fully experience and assimilate disappointment in me. It was only through experiencing my limitations, my inability to fulfill his intense longing for reunion with his father that he could gradually accept his own limitations and finally relinquish the wish to constantly chase after but always deny the death of his father. In the termination and post-termination phases, he had to experience me fully within the limitations of reality in order eventually to fully respond to the treatment as a success.

Mr. C had protested in the termination phase, "No way!" at the idea of becoming a better therapist to himself than I was. A few months after the end of treatment he wrote a letter about a puzzling piece of his history that he solved through working on a dream and then confirmed with his only surviving relative. He learned that, as an infant, he had been shipped out to his grandmother for a few months while his parents took an extended trip to Europe. "In the past I would have used the discovery to lord it over you, to exclaim that I could do something you couldn't do. But I don't feel that way. I am enormously grateful for the work we did together and for you equipping and allowing me to keep going. It took the full experience of our good-bye to access all the earlier good-byes."

Mrs. T had worked hard on a temptation to keep her analysis as a secret affair, an experience of acknowledging her own wishes and desires that she could not share with anyone other than the analyst. During the termination phase she had increasingly opened her heart to her husband, and he had been able to respond with greater involvement and understanding. A year later, Mrs. T wrote that everything was going well. She sent me a copy of a recently published story, with a note to say that she wanted to share her good feelings at this accomplishment. The story was in the form of an old woman's reminiscence about keeping secrets throughout her life. The bittersweet treatment of this theme represented a further reworking of Mrs. T's lifelong conflicts, transformed and integrated in a creative product that gave her new perspectives and expressive channels. The old woman in Mrs. T's last story tells her granddaughter that "secrets may be fun to make up but feel even better shared."

How Do Therapists React after Treatment?

As they approach termination, many patients worry that they will be forgotten once they stop. A tiny percentage of therapists avoid the feelings around goodbyes by changing the relationship with their patients, even marrying former patients. A larger number go to the other extreme, maintaining a reserved, even artificially cold demeanor when they happen to meet a former patient. We have heard of many instances where patients were puzzled and deeply hurt by this stance.

Most therapists grapple alone with their deep feelings on saying good-bye to a person with whom they have shared a unique, intimate, and often long relationship. This is intrinsically unlike ordinary partings. Most people may share feelings, reminisce about the person who is leaving, contact the absent one for news, or seek news from a third party. I said goodbye to George, a guitar-playing adolescent, over thirty years before publishing the first edition of this book. When we first wrote this chapter, he would have been a middle-aged man of fifty-one, and I have no idea about his subsequent life. As with all child and adolescent patients, I probably would not recognize him if we chanced to meet.

One way of dealing with feelings of sadness and loss is to institute formal follow-up.[1] In a 1997 paper, we suggested that analyst-initiated post-termination contact may be used to maintain the delusion of omnipotence.[2] Rather than leaving the initiative with the patient, where we feel it belongs, it could represent a radical change of stance and might disrupt the patient's independent progression. Instead of generating a rule, we have opted to tell patients at some point during the termination phase that we are always interested to hear about their lives, and about any and all kinds of news, as we wish them well going forward. We offer the possibility of one session a year at no charge, should they ever wish to meet. As we describe below, there have been many varieties of response to that invitation.

What Are Some Other Kinds of Post-Termination Contact after Child and Adolescent Treatments?

In child and adolescent treatment, we have found that if we work with the parents throughout and include them in the termination process, parents often contact therapists after the end of treatment for a variety of reasons.[3] These range from "running something by the therapist" consultations, to sharing news, to helping negotiate developmental transitions, to restarting treatment because something from inside or outside has overwhelmed the family's and patient's ability to handle it. Sometimes long-term follow-up comes from parents rather than the now-adult patient because they are concerned or feel a need to share feelings with the child's former therapist.

Occasionally, a parent shows empathy during the termination phase for the therapist's loss when treatment finishes. This seems to be due to our having succeeded in reassuring the parents that they are indeed the most important people to the child and that we are not competing with them. These parents then feel they can securely share the child with the analyst, as we saw with Kyla's mother.

Kyla started treatment as a violently aggressive preschooler and finished successfully at the age of seven. Much of the parent work addressed the divorced parents' valuing of themselves and how to help their child with loyalty conflicts between their very different parenting styles. Several months after therapy ended, Kyla's mother phoned me "because I knew you would so appreciate this." She described coming home from work and snapping angrily at Kyla. Later she apologized and explained to the child in some detail about her sense that she was taking something out on Kyla that really belonged in another situation. Uncertain about whether this concept was getting across, she asked Kyla, only to be met with a big grin and the remark, "Of course I understand how people sometimes do that, why do you think I went to my therapist for so long?"

Jane ended her analysis at twenty-one after five years of work on her suicide attempts. Work with her parents ended at the same time. In the four or five years afterward, I received occasional notes from Jane about important developments—her marriage, her first publication, the births of her children. There had been no news for twelve years when Jane called me for an appointment, saying that she had fallen into a terrible, suicidal depression.

When she was feeling hopeless, her mother had reminded her of how I had talked about monitoring her internal images of me and the treatment. When Jane saw that she had lost her sense of me as a benign, loving internal resource, she realized that she was killing off something important inside herself, and that this was a real danger signal. Jane and her mother were able to use tools from the adolescent treatment to deal with a current adult crisis. Due to the parent work during Jane's therapy, Jane's mother kept the image of me alive inside even when Jane could not.

What Are Other Ways Adults Make Contact after Therapy?

We saw above that letters and emails, especially those written soon after ending, are common post-termination contacts. Sometimes therapists are included in the email list for an annual holiday letter. Former adult patients may come for brief consultations around transitions in their lives, such as marriage, pregnancy, parenthood, illness, and so forth.

Mr. U had completed a successful treatment. I had not heard from him for many years when he called and asked if he could see me to discuss some concerns about change of career. He had done extremely well, his children were grown, and he was looking for something more challenging. As we talked, however, he revealed his main underlying reason for seeking a meeting. He had met a woman at work; he was smitten and sorely tempted to start an affair.

What emerged over a few sessions were old themes, reanimated by his developmental passage into middle age and his children leaving home. We revisited old feelings about transitions and abandonment. He realized then that he was feeling useless, unappreciated, and of little value to his family, as he had when his younger brother was born. The memories, insights, and subsequent resolution of his current conflict came quite easily, mostly through his own efforts. "I know I figured most of this out myself; there are times when your presence in my mind is enough. This time I think I needed to be in the room with you, with your presence helping me. I remember how I was so angry with you at the end of my treatment when you refused to become my best friend. Now I truly appreciate why you didn't, because now you are always there as a resource for me."

Former patients may get in touch when they are worried about a family member, especially their own children. As with Mr. U, they feel we are there as a resource for them but also sometimes for someone else. This may be a request simply for a referral, but often they specify their wish for us in particular because we will understand the ramifications of the situation.

Many years earlier I had treated a young woman for a severe eating disorder. Her symptoms resolved and she did well in college, living independently and having an active social life. She finished treatment after graduation, married a successful young man, and sent me notes when she had children. I had not heard from her for years when she called in great distress about one of her children. Mrs. R described her anguish over her daughter's eating disorder. Her daughter had gone to a prestigious distant university, and Mrs. R wanted a referral in that city.

Mrs. R was very upset and talked with me at length about her daughter's situation, but also about her own feelings and shock, since she felt she had truly left her original problem behind her. Her daughter, Grace, was denying the visible signs of her illness and refusing the idea of therapy. Mrs. R had never made a secret of her former difficulties, and after talking with me and revisiting some of the issues, she was able to talk with Grace from a position of emotional knowledge and strength. She said to Grace, "I know this is very hard, and it feels like not eating is the whole world. But that is a death. We are people who choose life, and I am going to get you the help you need." With my encouragement, Mrs. R and her husband brought Grace back home for medical treatment by familiar doctors, and she accepted a referral for an intensive psychotherapy.

Mrs. R asked if I would treat her daughter, since I had succeeded with her and she trusted me. I said I thought it would be better for Grace to have her own therapist, and I would stay available at this difficult time for Mrs. R.

Do Adult Patients Ever Resume Treatment with the Same Therapist?

An important measure of the solidity and depth of work in a treatment is patients' capacity to return without shame, guilt, or reproach to see the therapist when they are concerned that they are running into difficulties. If they reenter therapy, work can proceed on the foundation of the strong positive working relationship established in the first treatment. Patient and analyst know each other very well, and the work is efficient and deep at the same time.

Mr. E, who had come into treatment because of recurring panic attacks and an inability to find support in his loveless marriage, finished his therapy with firmly consolidated good feelings about himself and increasing reliance on a growing network of friends who shared his interests. Five years after the end of his long treatment, he called, saying that things were generally going well but he had a few issues to deal with. He wanted to see me "for as long as it takes to figure this out."

It is interesting to note that Mr. E, for reasons of cultural background and personality, had originally thought of therapy as something deeply shameful, indicative of weakness, femininity, and instability. By the time we finished our earlier work, his attitude was very different. He was an engineer, and he thought pragmatically that it made no sense to neglect a structure as complex as a human being. When he returned, there was no sign of embarrassment, disappointment, or feelings about failure on anyone's part. He described our renewed work as a "tune-up."

Mr. E had continued his loving relationship with the woman he had met near the end of our first period of work. They basically lived together while retaining separate homes. She was pressing for marriage, but for some reason he couldn't decide. "This feels like some old problem, so I thought I'd better come see you."

Faced with the intensity of his good feelings at the prospect of a second marriage, he found it difficult to hold on to his open-system functioning. He briefly fell back on old, closed-system, omnipotent ideas of placating his mother and defeating his pleasure-loving father by denying himself. "I guess it wasn't so much a tune-up I needed as a top-up. I have a leak in the system, and the good stuff we did and that I learned here seems to slowly drain out until it reaches the line. Then I have to come in and top up."

We noted earlier that some people take a long time to develop, consolidate, and integrate open-system functioning. Others, like Mr. E, seem to benefit from periodic revisiting of their alternatives.

Mr. Q had worked very hard and successfully on his rage and excited plans for revenge in his earlier treatment. He had married and had children. His wife then plunged into a serious depression, which did not seem to respond to either medication or therapy. He first contacted me for some suggestions about that situation, which was making him feel helpless. He then said that he really should come in himself, since he had begun feeling surges of frustrated fury at his wife, and he was worried that he would actually do something harmful to the family.

In the termination phase, we not only talk in general about post-termination phenomena but also anticipate with patients their particular vulnerabilities, for instance, Mr. Q's propensity for violent solutions. This is part of encompassing the reality that closed-system reactions never are truly eliminated. When Mr. Q resumed therapy, he remembered that we had talked about his potential to react this way to helpless frustration. It comforted him that we shared the understanding that, even in the midst of a rage, he needn't act on it but had another choice. He could call me, and we would figure out an alternative solution, as we had done many times before.

What Is the Impact of Post-Termination Contact on the Therapist?

We described earlier the important work in the pretermination and termination phases on differentiating disappointment of omnipotent magical wishes and the genuine and inevitable confrontation with the reality limitations of the therapist and the therapy, as well as of the patient. This helps patients return for consultation or renewed treatment without feelings of failure, shame, or blame.

Just as the patient has to distinguish between omnipotent and realistic goals, so does the therapist. It helps us assess the results of treatment clear-sightedly, without extremes of glory or abject failure. When we can achieve that open-system reality perspective, we can accept the need for further treatment comfortably.

We have noted that there is a difference between the criteria for beginning a termination phase and the goals of treatment. But delineating the goals of treatment is itself not that simple. In a literature review, we concluded that the vast array of suggested treatment goals varies wildly in the level of abstraction, in the degree to which they are theory-based, and in the extent to which they are overly pessimistic or overly optimistic. "Both within analysis and in the area of outcome research in general, there is an absence of consensus about what constitutes mental health and consequently how changes resulting from therapy are to be evaluated." [4]

In our new model of termination, we set the goals of treatment in terms of mastery of open-system therapeutic alliance tasks in order to restore the patient's capacity to choose how they want to respond to life's challenges. This is the overarching goal of therapy, worked on from the first phone call through the subsequent phases of treatment. The restoration of this capacity is assessed again in the post-termination phase. In the cases described in this book, each person was able to exercise their choice to find an alternative to the closed-system omnipotent solution that had been the predominant system of self-regulation accessible when treatment started. Contacting the therapist again because of difficulties is in itself an open-system act, demonstrating the exercise of the capacity to choose to take good care of oneself.

Knowing this helps therapists resist the pull to masochistic feelings of failure and depression when patients seem to relapse. Mental health professionals have a high rate of burnout and suicide. We think that recasting the goals of treatment in terms of restoration to the capacity to choose between two systems of self-regulation has a profound impact on how therapists can see their work.[5] Every interaction with patients generates data for assessing progress on this dimension of change. Having a choice is something that every patient can understand, first as a goal, gradually as an experience, and both are shared with the therapist, no matter what the theoretical orientation. This goal touches on profound human issues but is not overambitious since the potential capacity for creating alternatives and making a genuine choice is there in all patients, young and old, and all therapists, throughout life.

Do Patients Contact Therapists after Treatment with Positive News?

If we have worked well with the patient, and if we have conducted the work with our full, expansive array of techniques relating to both closed- and open-system functioning, and if we have shared a growth-enhancing good ending with the patient, then they are likely to want to share good news. This expression of open-system love from patients of all ages, including their parents, is another positive outcome of therapy.

Robert began analysis at three, having no speech and with a diagnosis of atypical or autistic development. He finished his treatment at seven years of age, good at swimming and competent self-regulation. I had not heard from the family since Robert's treatment had ended thirty years earlier. His parents saw a notice of a conference at the center where he had been treated, with my name featured as a speaker. Robert's mother left the following letter: "The reason I wanted to write to you for so long was to say that things have turned out so well for Robert." She described his school career, with success in academics and with friends, and his constructive and explorative adolescence. "He loved university, where he also met his future wife." She said he had done very well and pursued a career as a professional. "He has plenty of work, is very good at it, and loves it. He is happily married with two children. He is an exceptionally gifted and good father, as well as an excellent cook! He stands six foot four inches, is very serious, and is occasionally tense. He is very self-aware and totally honest about himself, he is affectionate and able to express his feelings. I think he is happy on the whole."

"I thought you'd like to know about him because you made a great contribution to his development by encouraging him to come out of his confines. Lastly I wanted to say that I too benefited from my visits to see you during a pretty difficult period in my life. For all this, many thanks."

Notes

1 Schacter 1990, 1992.

2 Novick, J. 1997.

3 K.K. Novick and J. Novick 2005.

4 Novick 1982, p. 357.

5 This is part of what encouraged us to describe our two-systems model in a slim volume called *Freedom To Choose: Two Systems of Self-Regulation* (Novick J. and Novick. K.K. 2016).

8

Final Thoughts

The questions that shaped this book came from students, patients, and colleagues as we have talked about termination over a span of sixty years. Our aim is not to give final answers but to engage readers in a dialogue around ending treatment, or indeed engaging with all changes and losses through life, in a mutually growth-enhancing rather than a traumatizing way. We think of this as working toward a "good goodbye" and have tried to describe both the difficulties and opportunities that arise within the context of ending treatment. We would like to leave readers with some general thoughts about ending.

- Termination issues should be engaged with from the first contact with patients. The sooner we become mindful of these issues, the more we can do to decrease the possibility of premature, bad endings and practice newfound strengths to ensure a good goodbye.

- Premature endings are frequent in all forms of psychological and medical treatment. They are wasteful and constitute a drain on scarce resources. Premature termination is a leading cause of frustration, despair, and burnout in the helping professions.

- Awareness of the frequency, dangers, impact, and causes of premature termination can equip therapists of all kinds to increase the rate of therapeutic success.

- Restoration of the capacity to choose between closed, self-destructive, and open, competent, and creative systems of self-regulation can be the overarching goal of all therapies, regardless of fundamental differences in theories of therapy.

- Therapeutic change does not stop with the end of treatment. A good goodbye enables patients to fruitfully continue the work of therapy independently for years afterward, as well as allowing for a return for additional work as needed without the burden of feelings of failure or blame.

- Termination of treatment is not death. But the achievement of a good goodbye equips patients (and therapists) with the emotional muscle to deal with the many expectable and unexpected losses, changes, transitions, and challenges through the life cycle.

We hope that this book stimulates readers to think about creating good goodbyes for themselves and their patients, and that the questions and our answers lead to further questions. Each treatment is co-created by the patient and clinician, and thus we cannot prescribe or make universal rules for the conduct of therapy. Rather, we hope that the guidelines we have described in this book help therapists increase their flexibility and expand the options for themselves and their patients to find their way safely and effectively through each treatment. You sent us your questions after the first edition, and we have answered them as best we can in this second one.

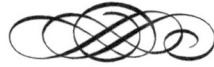

Appendix

There are several themes that thread through this volume and serve as the conceptual bases for our ideas about ending treatment. We have described them in three separate summary tables for ease of understanding, but the ideas intersect and relate to each other at many levels, so the tables should also be read together.

First is the model of Two Systems of Self-Regulation (Table 1), a way of thinking about the choices available to everyone at each time in life, as we work to grapple with life's challenges and maintain feeling good and safe. We consider that these choices are also woven into the fabric of the therapeutic relationship and the goals of treatment. Here we offer a summary table of the two-systems model, referencing the challenges at each particular phase of development and describing two types of possible responses. A more detailed description of the operation of two systems at each stage of development and throughout treatment can be found in our 2016 book *Freedom to Choose: Two Systems of Self-Regulation.*

Second is thinking about the importance of the therapeutic alliance (Table 2) to the experience and outcome of treatment. As an essential component of the therapeutic relationship at the heart of the endeavor, it demands participation by all parties. Our model of the therapeutic alliance is constructed in terms of tasks for patients, therapists, and significant others, with different elements highlighted at different phases of treatment. The table of therapeutic alliance tasks offers a summary. Our extensive writings on this topic offer more detail (see, for instance, Novick & Novick 1998, 2000, 2005, 2016).

Last, as we have described throughout this volume, we look at how a good goodbye in therapy resonates through the rest of life. We have discussed what may threaten a treatment at various junctures and what can support or rescue the process. The table of Risks/Obstacles and Protective Factors/Techniques (Table 3) summarizes our understanding.

We hope you find them helpful.

Table 1. Two Systems of Self-Regulation

Phase Challenge	Open, Adaptive, Competent Response	Closed, Omnipotent, Sadomasochistic Response
For parents during pregnancy *Parental helplessness re: physical changes, intactness and safety of baby*	Helplessness evokes parents' finding areas of realistic effectiveness and sources of support. Conscious planning to avoid repetition of own negative infantile experience.	Helplessness leads to parental fantasy of baby as controller, devourer, savior. Transference to baby from old relationships; intergenerational transmission of trauma/pathology. Externalization of devalued/feared/wished for aspects of self on to baby.
Infancy *Infant's failure to evoke needed response. Transient parental loss of attunement*	Mismatch followed by repair. This is root of positive feelings of competence, effectance, and reality-based self-regard. Positive feelings instigate and represent effectance and basic object tie. **Signs** include predominance of positive affect, secure attachment, psychophysiological harmony, empathy.	Parent fails child and infant is left in helpless rage, frustration, and traumatic overwhelming. Turn away from reality and competence. Reliance on magical controls. Attachment through pain. **Symptoms** may include gaze aversion, failure to thrive, hairpulling, head-banging, biting.
Toddlerhood *Exploration, independence, and assertion frustrated*	Child's aggression is absorbed in constancy of parental love. Exploration and assertion protected and enjoyed. Autonomy/separateness and independence a source of pride, with positive attachment strengthened at new level. Ambivalence tolerated, aggression increasingly separated from assertion. Anger and aggressive impulses a useful signal, calling into play ego capacities and realistic use of object. **Signs** include preponderance of joy, swift recovery from negative affects, capacity to accept help to negotiate resolution of conflicts, empathy, concern for others.	Assertion defined as aggression, parents helpless to absorb aggression, modulate excitement. Assertion becomes aggression becomes sadism. Intensity of feelings conflated with reality. Separation and separateness experienced as attack. Self-esteem derived from control of others. Identification with parental externalizations. **Symptoms** may include rages, sleep disturbances, separation problems, attacking self or others, interference with development of speech, toilet mastery, bodily control, mastery of feelings (tantrums, inconsolability).

Preschool *Reality of gender and generational differences (exclusion from adult activities)*	Turn to reality gratifications, internal sources of self-esteem. Development of autonomous conscience with both affirming and prohibiting characteristics, open to reality corrections. **Signs** include curiosity in service of growing reality sense, development of independent friendships, capacity to use adults as resources, tolerance of mixed feelings.	Child responds to trauma from overwhelming experiences (primal scene, frightening films, TV, etc) by sexualization, denial, and externalization. Parental collusion with child's wishes promotes formation of omnipotent delusion. Sadomasochistic beating fantasy organizes conscience, which is tyrannical, divorced from reality, unmodified by experience. **Symptoms** include persistence of earlier problems, inability to give up transitional object, bossiness and controlling behavior, provoking attack, obsessional rituals, bedwetting, ego constriction.
Schoolage *Negotiate rules, rewards, demands, and controls of external world.*	Good feelings from image of self as competent, effective, capable of learning, playing, negotiating, socializing, controlling self, and changing. **Signs** include successful mastery of impulses, tolerance of not knowing, development of complex relationships, capacity for pleasure in work and play.	Self-esteem based mainly on belief in control of others; Real talents and capacities co-opted to maintain delusional image of omnipotent self (entitlement, exception). **Symptoms** include persistence of earlier problems, intensification of obsessional rituals alternating with wild, "hyper," anxiety-driven behavior, lack of pleasure in real achievements, perfectionism, learning problems, bullying, victimization, inability to play, social isolation.
Adolescence *Real changes in body, mind, and social expectations.*	Ownership of mature sexual body. Consolidation of gender identity. Realistic self- and object-representations. Integration of pleasure, reality, and growth principles. **Signs** include pleasure in appearance and functioning of body, increase in capacity to parent self, constant relationships with peers and adults.	Maintenance of omnipotent beliefs by means of increasingly desperate self-destructive actions. **Symptoms** include pathological use of the body (eating disorders, self-mutilation, suicide, substance abuse, rapid repeat pregnancy, promiscuity), addiction, bullying, delinquency, depression, personality fragmentation, low achievement, grandiosity, social isolation.

(Continued)

Table 1. (Continued)

	Signs	Symptoms
Young Adulthood *Engaging with the reality of internal needs and external demands to find partner and career*	Using emotional muscles to tolerate risks and stresses of life choices; working on enhancing skills for life and work. **Signs** include managing the experience of loneliness, consolidating internalization of parenting functions, progressing in work life, taking pleasure in progressive functioning.	Resisting change, denying time, avoiding life tasks. **Symptoms** include "failure to launch"; recourse to drugs, promiscuity, porn addictions; adherence to extremist philosophies or groups; shallow relationships.
Adulthood *Creativity and generativity beyond oneself (parenthood)*	Engaging with the reality of growth, transformation, limitations, tolerating uncertainty; patience, tolerance, perseverance, altruism, flexibility; ownership of actions and self. **Signs** include stability of relationships and work life; dependable conscience and internally consistent behavior choices; pleasure in real satisfactions.	Rigidity, harshness, perfectionism; black-and-white thinking; authoritarianism, externalization of blame and responsibility. **Symptoms** include sadomasochistic relationships within family or work; delinquency or criminality; intolerance and tendency to conspiracy theories.
Middle Age *Change and transience; mortality*	Pleasure from realistic assessment of self and others; acceptance of mortality with enjoyment of time left. **Signs** include continuing creativity in new endeavors or interests; mentorship; re-ordering priorities to reflect reality.	Decreased tolerance, increased rigidity; denial of change and death; rage and blame at externalized foci. Search for rescue and respite in sadomasochistic enthrallment to outside figures. **Symptoms** include addictions, fad dieting, fanatical exercise, pursuit of cosmetic surgery, sudden affairs, precipitate divorce; increased denial, externalization and projection.
Old Age *Physical decline; mortality*	Pleasure in remaining capacities, in a life well-lived, ongoing shared pleasures; transformation of relationships. **Signs** include sharing experience and skills; making reparations where needed; acceptance of new configuration of powers between generations and role transformation with adult children.	Bitterness, despair, denial; externalization of blame and criticism; entitlement. **Symptoms** include destructive rage at younger people; abdication of responsibility; rudeness, prejudice, and rejection of appropriate help.

Table 2. Therapeutic Alliance Tasks through Treatment Phases

	Evaluation/ Exploratory	Recommendation	Beginning	Middle	Pretermination	Termination	Post-termination
Patient	Bring material; Engage in transformation tasks	Engage in setting goals	Being with therapist	Working together with therapist	Putting insights into action; Independent therapeutic work; Maintain progressive momentum	Setting aside omnipotent beliefs; Internalization of alliance; Mourning	Use alliance skills for living and creativity
Therapist	Initiate transformations of: Self-help to joint work; Chaos to order and meaning; Fantasies to realistic goals; External complaints to internal conflicts; Despair to hope; Helplessness to competence; Guilt to usable concern; Resist urgency	Articulate goals; Introduce working arrangements; Develop treatment plan	Feeling with the patient	Maximum use of ego functions	Allow for patient's independent therapeutic work	Allow patient's mourning; Deal with own loss; Analyze to end	Stay available as therapist
Significant Others/ Parents	Engage in and allow transformations	Endorse patient decisions	Allow the "being with"	Allow for individuation or psychological separateness	Enjoy and validate progression	Mourning loss of therapy; Internalization of alliance; Consolidation in phase of parenthood	Allow continued growth; Grow with patient
Relevant emotional muscle	Courage	Hope	Patience	Persistence	Tolerate painful feelings	Embrace full range of feelings	Holding on to gains

Table 3. A Good Goodbye: Risks/Obstacles and Protective Factors/Techniques through Treatment Phases

	Evaluation/Exploration	Beginning	Middle	Pretermination	Termination	Post-termination
Risks for premature termination from patient	Refusal of recommendation; Ghosting; Indecisiveness.	Denial of positive feelings and missing; Sadomasochistic power relationship.	Resistance to working together; Externalizations; Collaboration arouses anxiety.	Termination is real and will be unbearable; Flight or stagnation.	Equation of termination with death or lifelong depression; Blocking out love; Leaving in anger.	A bad goodbye leads to inability to continue growth.
Protective factors in patient	Pain from symptoms; Engagement with therapeutic alliance (TA) transformations; Acceptance of working arrangements.	Sees alternatives; Wish for more open-system functioning.	Pleasure in collaboration; Increased mastery and symptom reduction.	Pleasure and pride in treatment accomplishments; Experience of difference between depression and mourning; Increased emotional muscle.	Repeated experience of regaining open-system equilibrium; Experience of sadness linked to love.	A good goodbye leads to continued growth and capacity to return without blame or shame.
What Therapists Can Do	Initiate transformations; Find past and current open-system functioning; Present and explain working arrangements; Learn history of separations and loss, espec. in late adolescence; Set joint goals for pleasure, good feelings, mastery, and growth; Take long enough to start therapeutic alliance.	Understand resistances and symptoms as solutions protecting against helplessness; Link to past capacities and begin to draw contrast with present; Articulate goal of more effective, less costly solutions. Introduce consideration of pleasure, reality, and growth.	See non-collaboration as protection against rejection and loss; Introduce idea of emotional muscle to tolerate loss; Articulate pleasure and efficacy of collaboration; Point out closed-system solutions won't disappear; Label closed-system solutions as addiction.	Interpret anxiety and depression around loss as reversion to closed-system solution; Continue to point out conflict between two systems; Help consolidate open-system solutions as alternative to premature ending.	Interpret dread of ending equated with depression; Underscore link of mourning with sadness and love; Address internalization and object constancy in mourning process; Face own fears of ending as loss; Work as therapist to the end.	Stay available as therapist; Open door to post-termination contact.

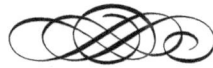

References

Ainsworth, M. (1985). Patterns of attachment. *Clinical Psychology, 38*(2), 27–29.

Ainsworth, M. (1991). Attachments and other affectional bonds across the life cycle. In C. M. Parkes & J. Stevenson (Eds.), *Attachment across the life cycle*. New York: Tavistock/Routledge.pp.33–51.

Ainsworth, M., Bell, S. M., & Stayton, D. J. (1991). Infant–mother attachment and social development: "Socialisation" as a product of reciprocal responsiveness to signals. In M. Woodhead & R. Carr (Eds.), *Becoming a person: Child development in social context*. Italy, Florence: Taylor & Francis/Routledge. pp.30–55.

Barratt, B. B. (1984). *Psychic reality and psychoanalytic knowing*. Hillsdale, NJ: Analytic Press.

Barrett, D., & Miller, J. (2024). Cultivating a culture of concern regarding confidentiality in writing about child and adolescent psychoanalysis. *The Psychoanalytic Study of the Child, 77*, 1–6.

Bergmann, M. (1988). On the fate of the intrapsychic image of the psychoanalyst after termination of the analysis. *The Psychoanalytic Study of the Child, 43*, 137–154.

Bergmann, M. (1997). Termination: The Achilles' heel of psychoanalytic technique. *Psychoanalytic Psychology, 14*, 163–174.

Bowlby, J. (1969). *Attachment and loss, vol. 1 attachment*. New York: Hogarth Press.

Bowlby, J. (1980). *Attachment and loss, vol. 3 sadness and depression*. London: Hogarth Press.

Coburn, W. J. (2000). The organizing forces of contemporary psychoanalysis: Reflections on nonlinear dynamic systems theory. *Psychoanalytic Psychology, 17*, 750–770.

Colarusso, C. (2024). A psychoanalytic retrospective: Thoughts on the essence of a happy and fulfilled life. *The Psychoanalytic Study of the Child, 77*(1), 143–155. https://doi.org/10.1080/00797308.2023.2264712

Colarusso, C., & Nemiroff, R. A. (1979). Some observations and hypotheses about the psychoanalytic theory of adult development. *American Journal of Psycho-analysis, 60*, 59.

Craige, H. (2002). Mourning analysis: The post-termination phase. *JAPA, 50*, 507–550.

Craige, H. (2009). Termination without fatality. *Psychoanalytic Inquiry, 29*, 101–116.

Donner, S. L. (2019). Review of Novick and Novick Freedom To Choose. *Journal of the American Psychoanalytic Association, 67*, 722–729.

Eagle, M. N. (2021). *Toward a unified psychoanalytic theory: Foundation in a revised and expanded ego psychology*. New York: Routledge.

Erikson, E. (1950). *Childhood and society*. New York: Norton.

Fehr, E. (2005). Cited in Amy Cunningham. *Scientific American Mind, 14*, 5, 6.

Ferenczi, S., & Rank, O. (1924). *The development of psychoanalysis*. New York: Dover.

Ferraro, F., & Garella, A. (2009). *Endings: On termination in psychoanalysis*. Trans. Dorothy L. Zinn. Contemporary Psychoanalysis Studies 10. New York: Rodopi.

Firestein, S. K. (1978). *Termination in psychoanalysis*. New York: International Universities Press.

Freud, A. (1965). Normality and pathology in childhood. *Writings, 6*, 3–273. New York: International Universities Press.

Freud, A. (1968 [1938]). The problem of training analysis. *Writings, 4*, 19, 407–421. New York: International Universities Press.

Freud, S. (1914). Remembering, repeating and working-through. *Standard Edition, 12*, 147–156. (1915).

Freud, S. (1918). From the history of an infantile neurosis. *S.E. 17*, 7–122.

Freud, S. (1926). Inhibitions, symptoms, and anxiety. *S.E. 20*, 77–175.

Freud, S. (1933). New introductory lectures on psycho-analysis. *S.E. 22*, 5–182.

Friedman, L. (1999). Why is reality a troubling concept? *JAPA, 47*, 401–425.

Fromm, E. (1947). *Escape from freedom*. New York: Farrar and Rinehart.

Goin, M. K., Yamamoto, J., & Silverman, J. (1965). Therapy congtruent with class-linked expectations. *Archives of General Psychiatry, 13*, 133–137.

Greenacre, P. (1971). Problems of training analysis. In *Emotional growth* (vol. 2, pp. 743–761). New York: International Universities Press.

Hanly, C. (1999). Subjectivity and objectivity in analysis. *Journal of the American Psychoanalytic Association, 47*, 427–444.

Hoffer, E. (1951). *The true believer*. New York: Harper.

Hughes, C. H. (1884). Borderland psychiatric records: Prodromal symptoms of psychical impairment. *Alienist and Neurologist, 5*, 85–91.

Hurry, A. (1998). Psychoanalysis and developmental therapy. In A. Hurry (Ed.), *Psychoanalysis and developmental therapy* (pp. 32–73). London: Karnac Books.

Kantrowitz, J. L. (2015). *Myths of termination: What patients can teach psychoanalysts about endings*. New York: Routledge.

King, P. (1980). The life cycle as indicated by the nature of the transference in the psychoanalysis of the middle-aged and elderly. *The International Journal of Psychoanalysis, 61*, 153–160.

Kinston, W., & Cohen, J. (1988). Primal repression and other states of mind. *Scandinavian Psychoanalytic Review, 11*, 81–105.

Lear, J. (2022). *Imagining the end: Mourning and ethical life*. Cambridge, MA: Belknap Press of Harvard University Press.

Levin, C. (1994). Containing the container: The structure of narcissistic fantasy and the problem of "primary undifferentiation." Unpublished manuscript.

Loewald, H. (1957). On the therapeutic action of psychoanalysis. In *Papers on psychoanalysis* (pp. 277–301). New Haven: Yale University Press.

Mayr, E. (1988). *Toward a new philosophy of biology*. Cambridge, MA: Harvard University Press.

Milner. M. (1950). Notes on the ending of an analysis. *The International Journal of Psychoanalysis, 31*, 191–193.

Modell, A. (1989). The psychoanalytic setting as a container of multiple levels of reality: A perspective on the theory of psychoanalytic treatment. *Psychoanalytic Inquiry, 9*, 67–87.

Norcross, J. C., Zimmerman, B. E., Greenberg, R. P., & Swift, J. K. (2017). Do all therapists do that when saying goodbye? A study of commonalities in termination behaviors. *Psychotherapy, 54*(1), 66–75. https://doi.org/10.1037/pst0000097

Novick, J. (1976). Termination of treatment in adolescence. *The Psychoanalytic Study of the Child, 31*, 389–414.

Novick, J. (1980). Negative therapeutic motivation and negative therapeutic alliance. *The Psychoanalytic Study of the Child, 5*, 299–320. (Later version in Novick and Novick 2007).

Novick, J. (1982). Termination: Themes and issues. *Psychoanalytic Inquiry, 2*, 329–365.

Novick, J. (1988). The timing of termination. *The International Review of Psycho-Analysis, 14*, 307–318.

Novick, J. (1997). Termination conceivable and inconceivable. *Psychoanalytic Psychology, 14*, 145–162.

Novick, J., Benson, R., & Rembar, J. (1981). Patterns of termination in an outpatient clinic for children and adolescents. *Journal of the American Academy of Child and Adolescent Psychiatry, 20*, 834–844.

Novick, J., & Novick, K. K. (1970). Projection and externalization. *The Psychoanalytic Study of the Child, 25*, 69–95. New York.

Novick, J., & Novick, K. K. (1992). Deciding on termination: The relevance of child and adolescent analytic experience to work with adults. In A. Schmukler (Ed.), *Saying goodbye* (pp. 285–304). London and Newyork: Routledge.

Novick, J., & Novick, K. K. (1994). Externalization as a pathological form of relating: The dynamic underpinnings of abuse. In A. Sugarman et al. (Ed.), *Victims of abuse* (pp. 45–68). Madison, CT: International Universities Press.

Novick, J., & Novick, K. K. (1996a). A developmental perspective on omnipotence. *Journal of Clinical Psychoanalysis, 5*, 129–173.

Novick, J., & Novick, K. K. (2007 [1996b]). *Fearful symmetry: The development and treatment of sadomasochism*. New York: Aronson (Rowman and Littlefield).

Novick, J., & Novick, K. K. (1999). Deferred action and recovered memory: The organization of memory in the reality of adolescence. *Child Analysis, 10*, 1–29.

Novick, J., & Novick, K. K. (2000). Love in the therapeutic alliance. *Journal of the American Psychoanalytic Association, 48*, 189–218.

Novick, J., & Novick, K. K. (2001). Two systems of self-regulation: Psychoanalytic approaches to the treatment of children and adolescents. *Special Issue Journal of Psychoanalytic Social Work, 8*, 95–122.

Novick, J., & Novick, K. K. (2003). Two systems of self-regulation and the differential application of psychoanalytic technique. *The American Journal of Psychoanalysis, 63,* 1–19.

Novick, J., & Novick, K. K. (2005). The superego and the two-systems model. *Psychological Inquiry, 24,* 232–256.

Novick, J., & Novick, K. K. (2016). *Freedom to choose: Two systems of self-regulation.* New York: IPBooks.

Novick, J., & Novick, K. K. (Eds.). (2022). *Adolescent casebook.* New York: IPBooks.

Novick, J., Urist, J., & Schneier, N. (1980). Patterns of unilateral and forced termination in an inpatient adolescent setting. I: Empirical results. Presented at the thirty-second annual meeting of the American Association Psychiatry Services for Children. New Orleans.

Novick, K. K., & Novick, J. (1998). An application of the concept of the therapeutic alliance to sadomasochistic pathology. *JAPA, 46,* 813–846.

Novick, K. K., & Novick, J. (2002). Reclaiming the land. *Psychoanalytic Psychology, 19,* 2, 348–377.

Novick, K. K., & Novick, J. (2010). *Emotional muscle: Strong parents, strong children.* Indiana: XLibris.

Novick, K. K., & Novick, J. (2005). *Working with parents makes therapy work.* New York: Aronson (Rowman and Littlefield).

Novick, K. K., & Novick, J. (2011). Building emotional muscle in children and parents. *The Psychoanalytic Study of the Child, 65,* 131–151.

Novick, K. K., & Novick, J. (2013). Concurrent work with parents of adolescent patients. *The Psychoanalytic Study of the Child, 67,* 103–136.

Novick, K. K., Novick, J., Barrett, D., & Barrett, T. (Eds.). (2020). *Parent work casebook.* New York: IPBooks.

Pinsky, E. (2002). Mortal gifts: A two-part essay on the therapist's mortality. *The Journal of the American Academy of Psychoanalysis, 30,* 173–204.

Rapaport, D., & Gill, M. M. (1959). The points of view and assumptions of metapsychology. In M. M. Gill. (Ed.), *The collected papers of David Rapaport* (pp. 795–811). New York: Basic Books. 1967.

Renik, O. (1993). Analytic interaction: Conceptualizing technique in light of the analyst's irreducible subjectivity. *Psychoanalytic Quarterly, 62,* 553–571.

Rokeach, M. (1951). Prejudice, concreteness of thinking, and reification of thinking. *Journal of Abnormal Psychology, 46,* 83–91.

Rokeach, M. (2015 [1960]). *The open and closed mind: Investigations into the nature of political systems and personality systems.* New York: Basic Books. Reprinted Martino Books: Connecticut.

Schacter, J. (1990). Post-termination patient-analyst contact I: Attitudes and experience; II: Impact on patient. *The International Journal of Psychoanalysis, 71,* 475–486.

Schacter, J. (1992). Concepts of termination and post-termination patient-analyst contact. *The International Journal of Psychoanalysis, 73,* 137–154.

Schlesinger, H. (2013 [2005]). *Endings and beginnings, second edition: On terminating psychotherapy and psychoanalysis.* New York: Routledge.

Schmukler, A. G. (Editor) (2019 [1992]). *Saying goodbye: A casebook of termination in child and adolescent analysis and therapy*. New York: Routledge.

Shore, A. (2002). Advances in neuropsychoanalysis, attachment theory, and trauma research: Implications for self psychology. *Psychoanalytic Inquiry, 22*, 433–484.

Sroufe, A. (2020). *A compelling idea: How we become the people we are*. Brandon, VT: Safer Society Press.

Steiner, J. (1993). *Psychic retreats*. London: Routledge.

Symposium. (1950). On the termination of analysis. *The International Journal of Psychoanalysis, 31*, 179–205.

Tessman, L. H. (2003). *The analyst's analyst within*. Hillsdale, NJ: The Analytic Press.

Tolpin, M. (2002). Chapter 11. Doing psychoanalysis of normal development: Forward edge transferences. *Progress in Self-Psychology, 18*, 167–190.

Tronick, E. Z., & Gianino, A. (1986). Interactive mismatch and repair. *Zero to Three, 6*, 1–6.

Von Bertalanffy, L. (1968). *General systems theory*. New York: Braziller.

Viorst, J. (1982). Experiences of loss at end of analysis: The analyst's response to termination. *Psychoanalytic Inquiry, 2*, 399–418.

Winnicott, D. W. (1949). Hate in the countertransference. In D. Goldman (Ed.), *In one's bones: The clinical genius of Winnicott* (pp. 15–24). Northvale, NJ: Aronson, 1993.

Young-Bruehl, E., & Bethelard, F. (1999). The hidden history of the ego instincts. *Psychoanalytic Review, 86*(6), 823–851.

Zhang, L., Levine, S., Dent, G., Zhan, Y., Xing, G., Okimoto, D., Gordon, M., Post, R., & Smith, M. 2002. Maternal deprivation increases cell death in the infant rat brain. *Brain Research, 133*, 1–11.

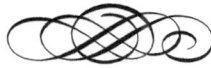

Index

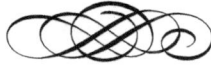

About the Authors

Jack Novick and Kerry Kelly Novick are life-cycle psychoanalysts on the faculties of numerous psychoanalytic centers. They trained at the Hampstead Clinic with Anna Freud in London, England, and at the British Psycho-Analytical Society and the Contemporary Freudian Society. In addition to their clinical work, they have been active in teaching, training, supervising, research, professional organizations, and the community. They joined other colleagues to found the award-winning nonprofit Allen Creek Preschool in Ann Arbor, Michigan, and the International Alliance for Psychoanalytic Schools. Separately and together, the Novicks have written extensively since the 1960s, with many book chapters and articles published in major professional journals. Their nine coauthored books have been translated into many languages.

www.ingramcontent.com/pod-product-compliance
Lightning Source LLC
Chambersburg PA
CBHW031137270326
41929CB00011B/1667